MW00596415

"You might be a Caregiver if...
your cup hath runneth over and you have too many
people and too many things to be thankful for!"

My cup hath indeed runneth over!

There is no way I could ever acknowledge all of the amazingly
wonderful, unique and "perfectly flawed" Caregivers that have
taught me, by example, along the way.

This book and dedication is essentially from "DOC" the "Defender of
Caregivers!" so it is lacking my own personal touch of dedications although
there are many that I would ad; my Little-Mom (Mother); my Children
(Stephen and Taylor); and my "Hood" (a neighborhood of giving-and
taking but most of all nurturing people).

The true Caregivers to whom I must dedicate this book are all the people
that I have worked with, served, fought, loved, laughed and cried with over
the past thirty years of my career as a professional (Nurture-"learned")
Caregiver and forty-plus years as a Nature-Caregiver ("Born"). Specifically
I want to thank the women (and a few men) at Seaford Center that taught
me the "Get Out of Bed and Go to Work!" philosophy that launched my
speaking career and gave DOC his voice.

I am forever grateful.
Thank YOU (all) for Caring!

Lon Kieffer, Caregiver, aka, DOC
The "Defender Of Caregivers!"

YOU MIGHT BE A CAREGIVER *if*

...you give yourself to *Others* and wonder what happened to *YOU!*

An original manuscript by:
LON KIEFFER, AKA, DOC, THE "DEFENDER OF CAREGIVERS"

CAREGIVERS GIVE THEMSELVES AND THEIR HEARTS TO OTHERS.
Learn how to protect yourself with Awareness and Acceptance
of who you TRULY are – *you might be a Caregiver!*

CONTENTS

Additional Reading

Appendix Section

Forward

As a nationally known speaker, author, and heart health authority I strive to find tools to help people learn how to prevent and control heart disease. Heart Disease is the number one killer of men and women. Stress is an independent risk factor for heart disease.

Over 50 million Americans are Caregivers for the adult population. The largest percent of Caregivers are women. The largest percent of people needing care will be women.

Women in this generation are dying unnecessarily. Since 1985 more women than men have died from heart disease. That's more than two decades.

As I search for tools that can be used during my speaking engagements and writings, how could I pass up the opportunity to seek information from Lon Kieffer, Caregiver, aka, DOC, the "Defender of Caregivers!"?

The strongest theme of Lon's book, "You might be a Caregiver if... you give yourself to Others then wonder what happened to YOU!" is his reminder to, "HONOR yourself as you Care for Others!"

One of the statements that grabbed hold of me and formed an immediate bond with Lon was this:

> You might be a NATURE Caregiver if...
> you don't need someone to tell you HOW to take care of yourself;
> you need someone to give you permission!

And, this book...

> You Might be a Caregiver if...
> you give yourself to Others then wonder
> what happened to YOU!

... is a must read for all of us.

With 78 million baby-boomers turning 65 years old in 2011 many of us find ourselves taking care of an aging parent, on top of raising our family and trying to create a future we can enjoy.

We can all learn more about what kind of Caregiver we are, as "DOC" shares with us case studies we can relate too.

What struck a major cord with me personally was...

> "You might be a Caregiver if...
> you feel guilty when you take care of yourself
> and angry when you don't"

As a woman on a mission to teach people how to control and prevent heart disease, I know how important it is to find time to take care of ourselves.

How do we do it? "DOC" shares with us that CHANGE or DIE is not about merely reorganizing or restructuring priorities; it's about challenging, inspiring and helping all of us to make the dramatic transformations necessary in any aspect of life – changes that are positive, attainable and absolutely vital.

DOC's own logo the protected heart – a heart with protective bands around it… sums it up as a heart that can give without being harmed. I find myself engulfed in learning Lon Kieffer's definitions of Caregivers and acronyms to live by.

Finally, Lon (DOC) shares wonderful quotes from people who have made a difference in this world. I find this particular quote helpful as people learn to love themselves more, by taking better care of their own hearts.

"To put the world right in order, we must first put the nation in order, to put the nation in order, we must first put the family in order, to put the family in order, we must first cultivate our personal life, we must first set our heart right." ~Confucius.

As a nationally known speaker, author of the auto-biographical book "Surviving", and a heart health authority I can say with confidence that Lon Kieffer's book, "You might be a Caregiver if… you give yourself to Others then wonder what happened to YOU!" is one positive step in the direction of setting your heart right!

Lois
Lois Trader, Speaker, Author, Heart Health Authority
www.loistrader.com

LON KIEFFER AND THE "DEFENDER" CONCEPT

My name is Lon Kieffer, and I....I am a Caregiver! You see it really cannot be said anymore plainly than that! I am a Caregiver. Even more so, I am a "Defender Of Caregivers!" *(more on that later)*

Yes, I am a father, a registered nurse, a healthcare executive, an internationally known speaker, "EnterTrainer" and consultant of common sense.... You can read about all of it on my website www.LonKieffer.com and in my blogs and other various self-promotional efforts and publications because lord knows... I have tried to get the word out there. But most of all....

..... I am a Caregiver!

And I say this knowing full well that you don't yet know what I mean in saying it; AND THAT IS VERY IMPORTANT because...

You Might be a Caregiver too!

In fact, I am betting that you ARE a Caregiver too! I am also betting that you not only don't yet truly know what I am talking about when I say it, I am betting you will argue with many of the conclusions I draw throughout this book even while agreeing with many of the things I have to say about you!

You see, even THAT is a Caregiver quality! You can see both; no, EVERY, side of an argument, so at times making a decision can be hard for you!

YOU MIGHT BE A CAREGIVER *if...*
YOU CAN MAKE LIFE AND DEATH DECISIONS WITH A SNAP OF THE FINGER, BUT YOU NEED 15 MINUTES WITH A DINNER MENU!

So, I am prepared to have you read this book saying to yourself, "Yep, that's me! I do that!" Or, "Oh, my God! That is soooo me!" and then when I tell you what it means you will say, "That's not me!"

Because.... You ARE a Caregiver! (or at least you might be?)

i

I am also prepared to DEFEND not only your right, but your need to do this… your right and your need to believe two diametrically opposed conclusions!

Why am I prepared to do this? Why am I prepared to ACCEPT and DEFEND YOU? Because… You ARE a Caregiver and I am DOC, the "Defender Of Caregivers!"

Before we go any further I have a confession to make… in addition to being a Caregiver I am also a frenetic speaker and story teller and… I CANNOT TELL A STORY WITHOUT JUMPING AROUND!

> *Seriously, writing this book is about killing me because I want to tell you the ENTIRE story NOW!*
>
> *Obviously that can't be done, things take time and follow a logical progression and order…but perhaps we can work something out?*
>
> *Here is an idea… at times in this book you will read about things like "Cognitive Distortions" but I may not have explained what they are yet… so feel free to jump forward to the Appendix section as needed and then back to pick up where you left off if I might mention something we haven't yet talked about.*
>
> *Or, you may read about things like "DOC-comments" (these are little side comments that DOC, the "Defender of Caregivers!" feels compelled to share even if they might seem out of place or order); or you may see what appear to be random Acronyms (words that are written like T.H.I.S.) when you see one of T.H.E.S.E. you can do one of two things; just accept the word as is and keep reading, or jump to the Chapter where we talk about Acronyms and Antagonyms to learn their underlying meaning (but keep in mind… that chapter is the big crescendo of this A.W.E.S.O.M.E. book!).*
>
> *But I promise… other than occasionally jumping around, it will all come together in the end.*

As a Caregiver you often find yourself employing a thought process called EMOTIONAL REASONING where you assume your FEELINGS validate your opinions or observations. "I feel it," thinks the Caregiver, "Therefore it must be true!"

As, DOC, the "Defender Of Caregivers!" it is my mandate to DEFEND you; even from yourself! Much like Professor Randy Pausch who, in his "Last Lecture", opened by saying, "My father always taught me… if there is an Elephant in the room, introduce him!" before telling everyone that he was dying of cancer. Thank you Randy Pausch for your "Last Lecture" and your living legacy!

Well, here is the Elephant in the room… this entire book and the "Defender Of Caregivers!" concept is based somewhat on my own EMOTIONAL REASONING and how strongly I FEEL about the observations I have made while working with and for the Caregiver's in my own personal and professional life. And here is the kicker... according to Dr. David Burns in his book "Feeling Good!" EMOTIONAL REASONING is a Cognitive Distortion (sic.. Caregiver Distortion #7)... it is a flawed way of thinking!

A.W.E.S.O.M.E!

This entire book and "Defender Of Caregiver!" concept is based on flawed thinking! Terrific! Aren't you glad you bought this book and wasted the last five minutes of your life to read this much only to find out it is based entirely on FEELings and not FACTS!?

Wait a minute... as is consistent with the mandate that I DEFEND Caregivers I, being a Caregiver, must also DEFEND myself and point out that dismissing the merits of my observations simply because I FEEL them strongly is an exercise in JUMPING TO CONCLUSIONS, where we draw conclusions (usually negative) from little (if any) evidence.

Well, guess what, JUMPING TO CONCLUSIONS is also a Cognitive Distortion in the eyes' of Dr. Burns (Caregiver Distortion #5) and in the world of two wrongs make a right; or in this case two distortions make a reality... we are going to proceed with our introduction of the "Defender Of Caregivers!" philosophy with one proviso...

YOU MIGHT BE A CAREGIVER *if...*
YOU ACCEPT THAT THIS BOOK (AND PHILOSOPHY) IS BASED
ON OBSERVATION (ANECDOTAL EVIDENCE)
RATHER THAN PURE SCIENCE YET YOU ARE INTERESTED IN
LEARNING MORE ANYWAY!

Now that we are done introducing and then ignoring elephants, let's get on with the core message of this book.

Once again, my name is Lon Kieffer and I am a Caregiver! I have had a 25 year career in healthcare and over that time, I began to notice certain common characteristics of the nurses, spouses, mothers, fathers, etc... responsible for providing Care to Others whether it be the professional or personal variety. As I began to crystallize these observations I found myself coming up with numerous... no hundreds (thousands?) of; You might be a Caregiver if... statements that highlighted a certain tendency or personality trait of Caregivers.

You might be a Caregiver *if...*
you agree to feed your neighbor's dog while they are on vacation yet forget to feed your own!

Yes, this originated from the Jeff Foxworthy "You might be a Redneck" jokes and was initially meant to simply be humorous. But as I began to share these statements with co-workers and co-Caregiverers (sorry I made that word up!), it began to snowball and these "You might be a Caregiver if..." statements began to take on a deeper meaning.

Further, as I was explaining and describing my observations of Caregivers and how so many of them seemed to be depleted rather than completed at the end of a long and honorable career I became convinced there had to be a common theme or personality trait among Caregivers.

I mean, it only makes sense, similar minds think and act alike, so why wouldn't there be a measurable, recognizable, even definable personality characteristic for Caregivers... well, it turns out there is and Myers-Briggs had already defined and described it for me....

So, that is when the journey really began to take off !

Being an "EnterTrainer!" (my first love next to writing) where I "teach through performance" I envisioned a one-man dramatic (and comedic) show called... "Defending the Caregiver!"

In "Defending the Caregiver!" I introduce my alter ego, DOC, the "Defender of Caregivers!" who always sees clearly! No distorted thinking for DOC... by the end of the show I realize that DOC and I are the same person... DOC is a more rested, more practical, more accepting version of myself...

Somewhere during my career, I became very aware that I had morphed into something I did not yet know that I had become (or even that I understood); I was a "Defender of Caregivers!"

Earlier in my administrative career, I would make rounds and wear my Caregiver patch on my sleeve (and my RN designee on my name badge). I thought it would give me credibility as I worked with and cared for the people in my organization; the people in my beds; the families in my lobby and visiting areas.

But you know what it really did? It confused the issue....It blurred the lines!

I learned that it was "not my job" to take Care of patients (insert your word of choice here), it was my job to take care of the people taking Care of patients (your word?)! I also learned I didn't have to Care FOR them; I only had to Care ABOUT them because my Caregivers were doing an amazing job Caring FOR them already.

So, I backed off and changed gears... it was NOT about Me!

Ironically, as I became AWARE of this and I began to ACCEPT, even embrace this philosophy, my career began to rise. I started to get awards and recognition; my speaking improved and had more passion and credibility... I had become the... DEFENDER OF CAREGIVERS!

When I began to concentrate on the Caregivers; the people that worked with me; the families that relied on us; the individuals doing the so called "heavy lifting" of both the physical and emotional variety; the Caregivers of both the professional and personal variety... everything got better!

The Care, the appreciation, the outcomes, even the bottom line; yes even the DOLLARS got better! In short... I decided my new role and job description would be "Defending the Caregiver!" and "my job" would be to provide perspective and support for Caregivers; I would become DOC!

The mission and goal of the "Defending the Caregiver!" philosophy is to provide a more rested, more practical, more accepting Caregiver in all of us simply through increased awareness and loving laughter... no therapy... just heightened awareness and loving laughter!

Loving laughter is, in my mind, the embodiment of ACCEPTANCE! If we can Love and Laugh together we have ACCEPTED one another wholly! (but not blindly) So, let's begin this journey and find out if;

You might be a Caregiver...?

Here is one final re-introduction of myself and this book, concept and philosophy....I am not a Doctor, I don't play one on TV program or on the Radio but I am DOC, the "Defender of Caregivers!" and, I....

I am... a Caregiver! and,

You might be a Caregiver too...

But even more importantly, I am DOC, the "Defender of Caregivers!" and,

You can be a "Defender of Caregivers!" too...

You Might Be A Caregiver *if*

...you give yourself to *Others* and wonder what happened to *YOU!*

CHAPTER 1

The World According to Myers-Briggs

R emember that elephant in the living room? Well, for this next section and chapter that elephant doesn't exist! Most of what you are about to read comes directly from Myers-Briggs, the world's most widely used personality assessment tool.

Of course, it is embellished and made more enjoyable to read by adding DOC's flair, but, in the end, it is the work of Myers-Briggs that we are discussing in this section. (For a more detailed explanation and description of Myers-Briggs please see the Appendix.)

The beauty in the work of Myers-Briggs, at least from DOC's perspective is how closely these researched and broadly accepted observations meshed with my own!

This epiphany was truly the inception of the "Defending The Caregiver!" philosophy and programs that are now approved nationally for continuing education for nurses by the American Nurse Credentialing Center (ANCC) at www.nursecredentialing.org.

The following is a mandatory disclosure:

This continuing nursing education activity was approved by the Delaware Nurses Association, an accredited approver by the American Nurses Credentialing Center's Commission on Accreditation.

Myers-Briggs has identified a personality type known as... drum roll please... "The Caregiver!" Now, before we slip deeply into the Myers-Briggs definition and description of "The Caregiver!" I want to share with you DOC's perspective: the entire concept behind "Defending The Caregiver!" is based solely in a desire to increase Awareness and pursue Acceptance.

Let's also take a brief side journey to explore what some of the world's greatest philosophers have to say about our personalities:

The great philosopher Popeye says; "I yam what I yam!"

Aristotle, a philosopher of some repute as well, says;
"We are what we repeatedly do!"

The French philosopher Renee' Descartes says; "I think (I am a
Caregiver) therefore I am (a Caregiver)!"

And finally;
DOC, a wanna-be philosopher says; "You are what you are
AND what you do! You are what you think of yourself!
You Might be a Caregiver!"

All of these great philosophers agree. Because of what or who you are, and HOW you THINK, and of what you do no matter who you do it for or where or why you do it for them!

"You might be a Caregiver!"

Later in this book we will discuss the DOC Philosophy of being a Caregiver by Nature (Popeye's version) or a Caregiver by Nurture (Aristotle's version)or a Virtual Caregiver (DOC's version), but that is for later in the book when we will reintroduce the elephant into the living room. For now, we are talking about accepted psychology-base Personality Typing.

So, if "You might be a Caregiver!" as defined by Myers-Briggs, DOC will teach you through increased Awareness to simply Accept it... and therefore reap the great benefits of a better understanding of yourself... so, take it away Isabel Briggs Myers.

*"Whatever the circumstances of your life,
the understanding of type can make your
perceptions clearer, your judgements sounder,
and your life closer to your heart's desire."*

~ Isabel Briggs Myers

A full explanation of how all this takes place is beyond the scope of this book, however if you would like to take a quick (10 minute) on-line version of the Myers-Briggs Typology Test visit:

www.humanmetrics.com/cgi-win/jtypes2.asp

The true and complete test takes several hours and must be administered by a certified professional. Once again, visit Appendix A of the book for a more detailed description and overall explanation of Myers-Briggs.

A PORTRAIT OF: THE CAREGIVER

(According to Myers-Briggs)

As a Caregiver, your primary mode of living is focused externally, where you deal with things according to how you feel about them, or how they fit in with your personal value system.

Your secondary mode of living is internal, where you take things in via your five senses in a literal, concrete fashion.

As a Caregiver you are a people person - you love people. You are warmly interested in others. You use your Sensing and Judging characteristics to gather specific, detailed information about others and turn this information into supportive judgments.

You want to like people, and have a special skill at bringing out the best in others. You are extremely good at reading others, and understanding their point of view. Your strong desire to be liked and for everything to be pleasant makes you highly supportive of others.

People like to be around you because you have a special gift of invariably making people feel good about themselves.

As a Caregiver you take your responsibilities very seriously, and are very dependable. You value security and stability, and have a strong focus on the details of life. You see before others do what needs to be done, and do whatever it takes to make sure that it gets done. You enjoy these Caregiver types of tasks, and are extremely good at them.

You are warm and energetic. You need approval from others to feel good about yourself!

You are hurt by indifference and don't understand unkindness. You are a very giving person. You get a lot of your personal satisfaction from the happiness of others. You want to be appreciated for who you are and what you give. You're very sensitive to others and freely give practical care. You are such a caring individual that you sometimes have a hard time seeing or accepting a difficult truth about someone you care about.

Because you are a people person and driven largely by your feelings, you are focused on reading other people and have a strong need to be liked, and to be in control. You are extremely good at reading others and often change your own manner to be more pleasing to whoever you're with at the moment.

The Caregiver's value system is defined externally. They usually have very well-formed ideas about the way things should be and are not shy about expressing these opinions. However, they weigh their values and morals against the world around them, rather than against an internal value system. They may have a strong moral code, but it is defined by the community that they live in, rather than by any strongly felt internal values.

Caregivers who have had the benefit of being raised and surrounded by a strong value system that is ethical and centered around genuine goodness will most likely be the kindest, most generous souls who will gladly give the shirts off of their backs without a second thought. For these individuals, the selfless quality of their personality type is genuine and pure. Caregivers who have not had the advantage of developing their own values by weighing them against a good external value system may develop very questionable values.

In such cases, the Caregiver most often genuinely believes in the integrity of their skewed value system (or distortion). They have no internal understanding of values to set them straight. In weighing their values against our society, they find plenty of support for whatever moral transgression they wish to justify.

This type of Caregiver is a dangerous person indeed and they are driven to control and manipulate others. However, they may lack Intuition preventing them from seeing the big picture. They're usually quite popular and good with people, and good at manipulating them. Caregivers are driven to manipulate others to achieve their own ends, yet they believe that they are following a solid moral code of conduct.

All Caregivers have a natural tendency to want to control their environment. Their dominant function demands structure and organization, and seeks closure. Caregivers are most comfortable with structured environments. They're not likely to enjoy having to do things which involve abstract, theoretical concepts or impersonal analysis. They do enjoy creating order and structure, and are very good at tasks which require these kinds of skills. Caregivers should be careful about controlling people in their lives who do not wish to be controlled.

You respect and believe in the laws and rules of authority, and believe that others should do so as well. You are traditional, and prefer to do things in the established way, rather than venturing into unchartered territory. Your need for security drives your ready acceptance and adherence to the policies of the established system. This tendency may cause you to sometimes blindly accept rules without questioning or understanding them.

A Caregiver who has developed in a less than ideal way may be prone to being quite insecure and focus all of their attention on pleasing others. He or she might also be very controlling, or overly sensitive, imagining bad intentions when there weren't any (Personalization - Caregiver Distortion #10).

Caregivers incorporate many of the traits that are associated with women in our society. However, male Caregivers will usually not appear feminine at all. On the contrary, Caregivers are typically quite conscious about gender roles and will be most comfortable playing a role that suits their gender in our society. Male Caregivers will be quite masculine (albeit sensitive when you get to know them), while female Caregivers will be very feminine.

Caregivers at their best are warm, sympathetic, helpful, cooperative, tactful, down-to-earth, practical, thorough, consistent, organized, enthusiastic and energetic. They enjoy tradition and security, and will seek stable lives that are rich in contact with friends and family.

* * *

So… are you ok with that? My guess is yes AND no!

There is a lot to like and admire in this description; there is also a little bit to maybe be aware of too. The description speaks to a tendency to get too wrapped up on certain aspects of our lives due to our personality and perhaps makes us vulnerable to distorted views on life.

Again, this is not overly scientific but while providing his "EnterTraining!" speaking services to a Healthcare client in Pittsburgh in April 2011 Lon, aka, DOC, the "Defender of Caregivers!" tried an experiment with 80-plus "Caregivers" that went as follows:

1. Using overhead projection he took them to the "Defender of Caregivers" website www.DefenderOfCaregivers.com.

2. He then took them to the "Continuing Education" tab and then to the LINK for: Take the Myers-Briggs Personality Test and Learn Your OWN Personality Type

3. For a shortcut you can just go here: www.humanmetrics.com/cgi-win/JTypes2.asp

4. He then had the group answer the 72 questions that make up the Personality Typology test. Again, they took this test as a group to determine their group personality.

And low and behold, as a group: the result was that they were… drum roll please… ACCOUNTANTS!

Just kidding, their collective personality was CAREGIVER.

Considering that Myers-Briggs has identified 16 Personality types and it is estimated that Caregiver personalities represents roughly 9 to 13 per cent of the population this public test was a bit of a risk.

But I was willing to take that risk to make a point. I don't have any statistics to offer to demonstrate this point, but the people with the Caregiver personality type are more likely to choose a profession such as healthcare that allows them to fully express their personality and personality type.

*   *   *

The official "Defender Of Caregivers!" spin on the Myers-Briggs Version of: The Caregiver! (an excerpt from: **"The Caregivers Dilemma: How to Care for Others without Losing Yourself!"** by Lon Kieffer, aka, DOC, the "Defender of Caregivers!") and foreward to the soon to be released book:

"The Distorted and Contorted Caregiver!"
Why they THINK they have to bend over backwards to help Others!

According to Myers-Briggs, the Caregiver personality derives satisfaction from pleasing others. At some level whether conscious or subconscious, whether admitted or denied, the Caregiver needs someone to care for in order to be satisfied themselves. As a result they may subconsciously hope the need for their Caregiving continues indefinitely and they may even resist the help or support they desperately need to survive. It's not that the Caregiver is unwilling to share the credit. The Caregiver is not looking for a great deal of accolades from others; their reward is within and based on how they value the satisfaction and services they provide to others. The Caregiver's Dilemma is if they accept too much help they risk diluting the self-satisfaction derived from the process of caregiving. Or worse, they may lose their role and a piece of their identity if the Caregiving relationship comes to an end entirely.

Part of the Caregiver's Dilemma is that much of this is subconscious. Saying this out loud or reading it here may even offend the Caregiver, as if their actions were selfish. They are not behaving selfishly; they are behaving naturally.

The Nature Caregiver suffers from this dilemma because they take satisfaction from pleasing others; the Nurture Caregiver suffers equally for the opposite reason; They don't take satisfaction from pleasing others yet they MUST do it anyway! Either way, the Caregiver cannot win!

The **Nature Caregiver** dismisses the service they provide (DISQUALIFYING THE POSITIVE, Caregiver Distortion #4) because it satisfies them so they reason subconsciously that their actions are selfish rather than virtuous; or expected rather than lovingly provided.

The **Nurture Caregiver** dismisses the service they provide (MAGNIFICATION OR MINIMIZATION, Caregiver Distortion #6 and ALL OR NOTHING THINKING, Caregiver Distortion #1) because they feel guilty for getting angry or frustrated since they provide these services out of an obligation rather than a sense of joy! They simultaneously MINIMIZE their services and accomplishments while self-determining through ALL OR NOTHING THINKING that they are somehow a bad person despite good deeds... in fact... they are also dabbling in LABELING and MISLABELING (Caregiver Distortion #9) when they determine they are themselves "BAD" for feeling this way.

So there you have it... the Nature Caregiver feels badly because they are acting Naturally and the Nurture Caregiver feels badly because they are acting Un-Naturally!

The idea behind this discussion is to allow the Caregiver to "see" this dynamic; to make them aware of it at a conscious level so that they can continue to be a Caregiver but stop denying themselves support (or self satisfaction). Again this is an internal dilemma; the Caregiver is not seeking approval or praise but internal worth based entirely on how they value what they have done for others. In the end, the only thing the Caregiver truly seeks from other people is acceptance; a belief that others "get them," that they understand. The Caregiver wants to be appreciated and understood! Often the Caregiver simply needs someone to hear and understand them; and nothing more. DOC, the "Defender of Caregivers!" was created for this purpose!

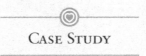

CASE STUDY

The case studies used in this book are real; and represent Caregivers that are active members of the "Defender of Caregivers!" Fan Club. Names have been changed as a courtesy to these amazing people.

Alice's Story:
The Professional Caregiver (Myers-Briggs)

Our base personality drives our actions. For "the Caregiver" this often means they pursue a career that will mesh with their base personality and the field of Nursing is a natural fit... but not always a healthy fit.

This Case is about Alice, a professional nurse; a nurse that came into the profession later in life after being a housewife, a vocation that I am certain made full use of her Caregiver Nature. As the Myers-Briggs portrait of "the Caregiver" would predict, Alice's home life was stable and loving; she had one child that she raised well. As her son grew up and became more independent, Alice started her nursing career in a nursing home. When her son was sent off to war she began to pursue more professional education to advance her nursing career. After his deployment, he remained active duty and the military moved him away from home.

Without her son to Care for, Alice concentrated even more on her career; always learning more in an effort to fulfill perceived and or actual needs within her Center. Eventually, she became renowned for her skill at healing and preventing wounds (decubitis ulcers). She also became known for volunteering to work split shifts on holidays to allow her co-workers time off with their families. She said, "Half my family is gone now, so I can work half a day (even though by tenure she could have been off) so you can spend half a day with your family!" Everything was great! She was fulfilled.

Then her husband got sick... out of the blue, he was diagnosed with terminal cancer. So now, our Professional Caregiver was also a Personal Caregiver and she was conflicted. Alice began

20

Caring for her husband AND Caring for her patients AND Caring for her co-workers… and quit Caring for herself.

YOU MIGHT BE A CAREGIVER IF…
YOU SOMETIMES HAVE TO CHOOSE BETWEEN CARING FOR THOSE YOU LOVE AND THOSE YOU LOVE TO CARE FOR!

For the first time in her life, Alice was relying on Others for help; she occasionally had to miss work because she was needed at home. The guilt she felt for leaning on her co-workers was obvious. She had no insight into the simple fact that this, for them, represented a rare opportunity to balance the pendulum of a relationship that up until now was always one-sided; Alice had always DONE for them and they could never do anything in return for Alice.

Eventually, with her husband in full decline he saw that she needed help and demanded she get help for "her" by accepting help with him. With the encouragement of her co-workers to "stay away" from work and concentrate on home, she reluctantly agreed to accept help. Ultimately, she agreed to place her husband in a hospice program. He was admitted on a Friday afternoon of a Holiday weekend. She was scheduled to work on Friday… and would then be off the next week to spend with her dying husband; but she refused to take off that Friday and ruin another co-worker's Holiday weekend. They all begged her to take off and she said, "No. He is doing great. He's stable. I will go spend the night with him after I get off!" Well, you know what happened. He died while she was at work, leaving her with guilt and feeling like she had failed him because she was not at his side. Instead of being able to celebrate her noble efforts and loving loyalty, she felt regret.

Today, she continues to work in the same nursing facility, lives in the same house, takes care of the same co-workers. She has even begun taking in borders, etc., to help financially stressed co-workers in transition.

Always the Caregiver; always the professional…

DOC Comments...

This is a classic example of the Myers-Briggs personality at play... a Caregiver by NATURE pursued Caregiving as a profession and, for the most part, was and is an engaged, healthy and committed yet well-rounded person. With the exception of the period in her life where she was conflicted by both the desire and the demand as a Caregiver to "choose between Caring for those she loved and those she loved to care for!" she was able to maintain a rational approach to life.

But during this time... she was hyper-stressed, contorted and distorted, and unable to consistently make decisions that would be, first and foremost, in her own best interests.

She had not lost HOPE; and she had already naturally established "VALUE Circles" but in this case she needed a DOC to apply the L.A.W. to her case and help her see this situation clearly and allow her to make the best decision to: HONOR herself as she Cared for Others!

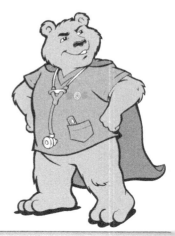

CHAPTER 2

The World According to Popeye!
(The NATURE Caregiver)

Let's start this next Chapter with an excerpt from the "Defender of Caregivers!" blog where, through the use of short stories and anecdotes, DOC shares lessons about the Caregiver's Dilemma and general principles about leadership and organizational development.

Please enjoy:

"Was Popeye the Sailor Man a Caregiver?"

(originally published July 8, 2010
at http://www.defenderofcaregivers.com/blog/?p=44

Popeye was famous for saying,

"I yam (am) what I yam (am)!"

Well, as a Caregiver, "you yare (are) what you yare (are)!"

And you yare (are) a Caregiver!

Once a Caregiver, always a Caregiver;

once a parent, always a parent!

Popeye, in my mind, was a Caregiver... he was always thinking of and out to save others! "There's women and infinks on that ship!" he would say, and then dive head first into the water without a thought for his own well being.

Popeye always sang this song (and "DOC" added a new ending):

I yam what I yam and I yam what I yam that I yam…

And I got a lotta muscle and I only gots one eye…

And I'll never hurt nobody's and I'll never tell a lie…

Top to me bottom and me bottom to me top…

That's the way it is 'til the day that I drop, what am I?

I yam what I yam"

… a Caregiver is what I yam! (DOC's addition!)

Here are some lessons Caregivers can learn from Popeye:

1. Love is blind! (Olive Oyl – "'nuff said!")

2. Spinach is good for you!

3. We can only be hurt by the ones we love! (Popeye's strength was no match for Olive Oyl, who frequently treated him badly despite his constant efforts to please her… sound familiar?)

Learn to enjoy the moments where YOUR Caregiver is showing! Popeye: "Here's me past record folks, which speaks for itself!" You are a Caregiver… that speaks for itself! Thanks for Caring!

* * *

In this Chapter we will explore the Nature Caregiver… people who are BORN into the role of the Caregiver.

According to testing roughly 9 to 13 percent of the population are true "Caregivers" (ESFJ) as defined by Myers-Briggs.

These Caring people will likely pursue careers and or relationships that allow their personality to flourish and develop. They are quite content in being the stronger, more stable, more energetic person in a relationship whether it is personal or professional.

So… then everything for them is hunky-dory, right?

They want to take care of Others and they find people that need to be taken care of so everything is perfect, right?

Not so fast… this group of people actually are very prone to the

Caregiver's Dilemma (where they lose their own identity and ability to Care first for themselves because they are stressed by Caring for Others) for the simple reason that they don't see a Dilemma!

That is, until it's too late!

Because this role comes so naturally to them they may be in a lifelong Caregiver relationship and not even know it... and no, I am not talking about garden variety Co-Dependency (that is someone else's book) where the person that is acting out is the "weak" link in the relationship (frankly, I would ask that you just accept that description because spending too much more time explaining it is a distraction from the point.. which is the Caregiver and this book is about THEM!)

The difference between Co-Dependency and the Caregiver's Dilemma is that with the Caregiver's Dilemma it is the so-called "strong" link in the relationship that is acting out! The Caregiver is the problem here... the person or persons they are Caring for is NOT the focus of this book.

They don't get a free pass as I realize there are people who demand more attention or Caregiving than should or could be expected; there are those who place Caregivers in impossible situations and circumstances... but again, this book is NOT about them!

This book is about the Caregiver!

And in this context it is the Caregiver that is the problem!

"How is that fair?" you ask. "The Caregiver is working their butt off to take care of someone else and you say THEY are the problem!"

> "Am I a bad person?" asked Sandra Bullock's character in the movie "The Blind Side"

> "You are a great person," says Tim McGraw, "Everything you do, you do for someone else!"

See, THAT is the problem with a NATURAL Caregiver... "EVERYTHING they do, they do for someone else!"

Aside from it being a little annoying (to Others), it must be exhausting to constantly do EVERYTHING for Others! But, according to the NATURAL Caregiver, NOT!

They are quite content with the fact that "everything they do, they do for someone else!"

You notice I keep writing that over and over and over again... well, it's because they keep doing it over and over and over again!

And all the while, just like Sandra Bullock in her Academy Award-winning portrayal of Leigh Anne Roberts Tuohy, the Caregiver ends up wondering, "Am I a bad person?"

And they wonder "Am I a bad person?" because it is never enough. They can never do enough for other people, so in some way they will always be left feeling inadequate.

Yet, because the Caregiver can go back to their Caregiving ways, because they can go back to what they enjoy, they don't truly have to be faced with answering their own question, and if they do it would go something like this...

> *Caregiver to self: "Am I a bad person?"*
>
> *Caregiver to self: "I am what I am!"*
>
> *DOC comment:*
>
> *"The NATURE Caregiver feels badly because
> they are acting naturally!"*

After this little dialogue, they then get back to being busy with their Caregiver duties and forget they even asked the question... that is until they face a set back or a temporary meltdown and they begin to doubt themselves all over again.

Or, the other scenario is that they are forced to stop being a Caregiver and only then do they realize that they have lost themselves.

The real challenge for the Caregiver is that they enjoy doing for others so they find it very hard to ever stop doing for others. They view themselves as the center of the universe, but not in a narcissisti way... they just have a need to do things for Others to please them... to please themselves!

Caregiver Vision

This is how the NATURAL Caregiver sees the world...

ESFJ is techno-speak for the combination of typology used by

Myers-Briggs to describe "the Caregiver, etc... so, ESFJ essentially means, Caregiver.

In this classic Schnellen Chart, the Caregiver sees themselves as being in the center of the world and they believe that "they are not happy unless those around them are happy!"

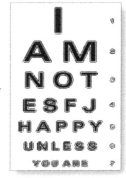

This view of the world is distorted by their NATURAL personality and their need to please others.

And this distorted vision becomes a MENTAL FILTER (Caregiver Distortion #3) that they process all information through in their daily lives.

Yet, they don't even know they are doing it...

> Glinda (a "good" Witch) in the Wizard of Oz:
> "Are you a good witch or a bad witch?"
>
> Dorothy: "Me? I'm not a witch at all!"

When I speak as DOC, I always ask my audiences; "How many of you are Natural Caregivers?"

You would be surprised at how many people respond: "Me? I'm not a Caregiver at all!"

Most of those who tell me they are not Caregivers "at all" are men; or women in non-clinical roles such as the business office or information technology.

I tell them that they all "might be" Caregivers whether they know it or not.

The only real question is whether they are Nature or Nurture Caregivers. Unlike Glinda's question to Dorothy, there is absolutely NO implication that there is such a thing as a Good Caregiver or a Bad Caregiver implied in this question.

The truth is... we are all BORN(E) Caregivers!

(NOTE: BORNE is a past participle of the word "bear" as in, to "hold up; support" but not BEAR as in DOC the bear who was BORN on the pages of this book!)

Whether it be that you are BORN into it by having a Natural Caregiver Personality or whether you are BORNE into it by having accepted (or inherited) a burden or responsibility to act as or become a Caregiver... you are a Caregiver!

You might be a Caregiver *if...*
you just want to help people (NATURE/Born)
or you have no choice
but to help people (NURTURE/Borne).

You might be a NATURE Caregiver *if...*
you don't need someone to tell you HOW
to take care of yourself
you need someone to give you permission!

DOC, the "Defender of Caregivers!" is here to give you permission to take Care of yourself.

I am here to tell you to HONOR yourself as you Care for Others!

Along the way I will offer you honesty and encouragement; I will offer Affirmations, Acronyms and Antagonyms too... sorry, I am just having fun now!

I hope you enjoy this journey because there are going to be times where you don't like what I have to say about you... but know this... I am in AWE of you!

Thank you for Caring!

You might be a NATURAL Born Caregiver!

28

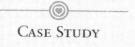

CASE STUDY

*The case studies used in this book are real; and represent Caregivers that are
active members of the "Defender of Caregivers!" Fan Club.
Names have been changed as a courtesy to these amazing people.*

Unlike other Caregiver-types, here we will offer two different
Case Studies because the NATURAL Caregiver Personality
expresses themselves in many different scenarios. One case is
not sufficient to begin to capture this phenomenon. Again, both
of these cases are actual and active members of the "Defender of
Caregivers!" Fan Club; any inaccuracies are unintentional and
a by-product of literary expediency or an effort to reflect the
true NATURE of the story yet provide a modicum of privacy and
plausible deniability for DOC, the author; their names have been
changed as a courtesy... but knowing them, they will probably
jump on-line and claim these descriptions as their own!

However, DOC encourages them NOT to!

Nancy's Story
The Serial Caregiver (NATURAL Caregiver)

The NATURAL Caregiver that is not fully aware of their
Natural personality can get caught up in a confusing world
where they continually and repeatedly – serially - seek
Caregiving opportunities. Some Caregivers coincidentally find
themselves in relationships where the Caregiver role evolves, uh;
naturally... they are called into duty. Others don't get that call
and they seek the role.

Nancy is a Natural Caregiver who found herself in young
adulthood unmarried and unfulfilled. By a twist of fate, she met
a quadriplegic man and fell in love quickly and married him.
For the next dozen or so years, she faithfully stood by him and
Cared for him until he tragically died. Nancy was at his bedside
and Cared for him until the end and even then, after he died,

she continued to Care for him and gave him a respectful funeral. After all, he had no family to speak of and it was up to her.

Once the tears and tributes were over, Nancy came to a realization; She was chronologically in her mid-30's yet she had no career, no family and her biggest skill and role in life, providing Care for her now-deceased husband, was no longer needed. She felt worthless.

Since she didn't know what else to do with her time and her talents, she volunteered at the health center, where she frequently took her former husband for therapy. There she met another man; also a quadriplegic, and again, she fell in love with him and was quickly married. Fifteen years later, she found herself at another funeral burying another man that she loved and had dutifully and lovingly Cared for.

Now in her late 40's and with her own health in decline due to an ignored and untreated condition of adult onset diabetes, she once again felt lost.

It was at approximately this time that she found the "Defender of Caregivers!" Group on Facebook. While I wish DOC could take credit for what happened over the next 18 months it is not my role to claim credit or imply causation... but I am re-telling the story accurately.

First, DOC "made her pay" for her laughter. DOC put up a post on Facebook poking fun at himself; here is that post:

You might be a (Male) Caregiver if...
YOU FIND YOURSELF SO BUSY THAT
YOU STAND WHILE YOU EAT
BUT SIT WHILE YOU PEE!

Nancy responded with; "LOL... too funny! DOC... YOU might be a Caregiver!"

In that moment of Loving Laughter, DOC realized that they had a connection; a shared sense of HUMOR (a Healthy

<u>U</u>nderstanding of a <u>M</u>oment <u>O</u>thers <u>R</u>ejected) and experiences and he made her pay for it...

DOC believes in making people pay for Laughter because it means something; shared laughter is an intense moment of mutual understanding and here is how he made her pay, "Nancy.... I believe that if I can't laugh at myself, I can't laugh at others; and Nancy, if you can't take Care of yourself, you can't take Care of Others. As payment for that laughter I want you to promise me you will go get your diabetes checked out!"

DOC began telling her to HONOR herself as she cared for others; DOC encouraged her to slow down on jumping into the next relationship and OPENLY suggested she ACCEPT her tendency to fall in love quickly and to learn how to LOVE herself first... when she said she didn't know how to do that DOC suggested that she PRACTICE, that she get a massage, have her nails done, go on a real vacation!

By virtue of her simple decision to join and interact with the "Defender of Caregivers!" Group, she had begun on her own to ENGAGE other Caregivers in Value based relationships...

On her own, she began to explore other aspects of her life that she had ignored previously. She began attending church and found a church with a strong musical base. Music was a strong and long-lost Love from her childhood. She met a man that was spiritual, musical and also... a NATURAL Caregiver who had recently become a widower of a woman he had not only Loved but Cared for. After almost a year (an eternity for both of them), they got married and are taking Care of each other.

Nancy satisfies her Caregiver needs by working as an in-home Caregiver for the Elderly.

DOC Comments...

The term Serial Caregiver is a term created and defined by DOC. You won't find it anywhere else! It may not even be a legitimate title or moniker, but I promise... I have seen it play out numerous times.

This is the DOC version of a phenomenon known as: The Florence Nightingale effect; a term used to describe a doctor's, nurse's or other caregiver's development of feelings for his/her patient. This effect causes a feeling much like infatuation, love or sexual attraction to come over the caregiver regarding a patient, even if very little communication or contact takes place outside of basic care. Feelings may fade once the patient recovers; in Nancy's case, her patients with permanent paralysis could never recover... her love never faded... she did.

Again, DOC is not taking credit for what happened, but it did happen after Nancy joined the "Defender of Caregivers" Group so... just sayin'
Not only did Nancy find DOC, she found herself and she found H.O.P.E.

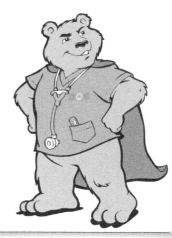

THE AMAZING CAREGIVER (NATURAL CAREGIVER)

The NATURAL Caregiver often "finds" himself or herself when they weren't even looking and then "loses" himself/herself when they were struggling for an identity. Finally he or she may only truly find themselves after and because they once were lost!

YOU MIGHT BE A CAREGIVER *if...* YOU BELIEVE THIS WOULD BE THE SONG/STORY OF YOUR AMAZING LIFE!

Amazing Grace
How sweet the sound
That saved a wretch like me
I once was lost
But now am found
Was blind but now I see

'Tis Grace that taught My heart to fear
And Grace my fears relieved
Now precious dear That Grace appear
The hour I first believed

When we've been there
Ten thousand years
Bright shining as a sun

We've no less days To sing God's praise
Than when we first begun

Amazing Grace
How sweet the sound
That saved a wretch like me
I once was lost
But now am found
Was blind but now I see

I once was lost
But, now, now I'm found
I once was blind
But, now, now I see

Janet had it all: a wonderful marriage, a successful business (two in fact) that she co-managed with her husband; a nice house; three beautiful kids. Her Caregiver tendencies began to show themselves early and drove much of her thinking processes in quite unnoticeable ways. She had a life-long dream to be a stay-at-home Mom so she could Care for and raise her three young children. Due to her driven devotion to family and business she and her husband achieved this goal and life was perfect.

Then, tragedy struck. A work-related accident put her husband in crisis with a tragic and horribly mis-diagnosed and then mis-managed spinal injury. After years in and out of hospitals, surgeries, infections, courses of over and mis-medicated medical management, her dream-husband was gone. Ultimately Janet and her kids found themselves living with a physically debilitated man with adult-onset bipolar disorder (stress or medicine induced?); chemical and alcohol dependency developed and he was physically and mentally abusive. Add to the equation the failure of their business ventures, and the financial ruination of the family home.

Throughout all of this, Janet stuck by her man! Every endeavor of her life revolved around being a better Caregiver, a better mother! She remained dedicated to her husband AND her children; she endured the physical and emotional abuse and held the family together.

After years of repeated strain, she herself began to falter. Her psyche was already damaged and now her physical health began to deteriorate as well. She developed Chronic Fatigue Syndrome, Conversion Disorder, Fybromyalgia (all classically "stress" disorders and all with alarmingly high incidences in the Caregiver community) and other medical problems that, in essence, did for her what she could not do for herself... these ailments forced her to stop acting out as a Caregiver!

Janet started to focus on her own health; not because she had a new awareness of the importance of it but because she had no choice! Today she says, "Ultimately, the only reason I was able to help myself was because I didn't know who I was anymore... I started to view myself as someone I didn't know... someone that needed my help!"

Janet ended her marriage and began to rebuild her life; she continues to suffer from guilt over "having failed" in her Caregiver duties and in her marriage. But wait a minute... there is a twist to all of this...

Just like the decline of her physical health forcing her to deal with her failing mental health, her husband forced her to deal with her failing marriage. That's right... after 20-plus years of devoted marriage and a decade of loyal Caregiving, HE LEFT HER for an old classmate he met on Facebook. A short time later, he came crawling back...but because of another amazing intervention Janet chose herself and her children over her husband, and refused to take him back.

What was this amazing intervention, you ask? It was that she naturally stumbled onto and into a V.A.L.U.E. Circle! Janet became a member of the "Defender Of Caregivers!" Group on Facebook and began to receive the "What's Up DOC!?" Newsletters (again, DOC is not claiming to be a miracle worker here... after all, Janet would not have found DOC if she had not already started this journey on her own... but DOC was there when she needed him/us... so, just sayin') and eventually, through the "Defender of Caregivers!" Group Page and Website Janet, met and began a relationship with Cheryl... it was a cross-country virtual relationship at first; but it was V.A.L.U.E. based!

Eventually they went on to meet and continue to have a relationship based on mutual understanding and Giving and Receiving V.A.L.U.E.

Today Janet is active in Yoga, which helps her physical and emotional pains and remains a very active member of the DOC Fan Club on Facebook.

UPDATE: *The very day that DOC reached out to Janet in order to establish some boundaries regarding the writing of this "Case Study," Janet received a panicked phone call from her ex-husband; a short time later, she received a phone call from one of her daughters and other friends seeking help for him. All of her emotions came back in a rush and she started to go to his aide... this literally was happening at the same time... she sent DOC a message that she would have to work on this project later because he needed her... but she reached out to Cheryl and within herself and instead of going to help him... she suggested they call 911 and she went to her Yoga class.. "It was the right thing to do, for me!" she said.*

DOC Comments...

Wow! Janet's story both scares and amazes me! Everything you have read is true but perhaps not entirely accurate; what I mean by that is in an attempt to tell this story quickly (in a certain amount of words as dictated by my editor) I have abbreviated it and cut some corners... but it is true.

The number and degree of Caregiver Distortions she was exhibiting and utilizing are simply too many to mention. Her entire life was judged and every decision based on the MENTAL FILTER (Caregiver Distortion #3) of her life as a Caregiver. She made NO decisions based on her own needs! Janet deserves all of the credit! DOC's role in this was very coincidental and I am concerned that the telling of this story implies or appears that he and I believe otherwise... we don't! But we are very glad to be here and that Janet and Cheryl found us! They created their own V.A.L.U.E. Circle; they provided one another H.O.P.E., the obeyed the L.A.W.

The pictures of Janet from her 48th Birthday when she THOUGHT (Distortedly) she was a happily married Caregiver to her 50th Birthday where she is acutely AWARE and ACCEPTING that she is a healthy-but-not-always-happy (a perfectly flawed individual) recovering Caregiver are simply amazing. She went from looking like a woman literally on the verge of major medical crisis to a beautiful and vibrant woman! She has been encouraged to write a book and I hope she will let DOC write the forward! Janet... you are AMAZING... once you were blind (distorted) but now you are found (you are AWARE)... at once you were blind but now you see (you ACCEPTED yourself)... you have GRACE!

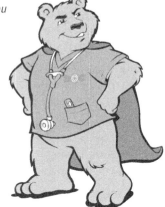

CHAPTER 3

The World According to Aristotle!

(The NURTURE Caregiver!)

"You are what you repeatedly do..."

~ Aristotle

E ven if you are NOT a Caregiver... and you don't want to be.. sooner or later, if you are thrust into the role, you become one! "You are what you repeatedly do!" says Aristotle

So, for you, being a Caregiver is a learned behavior. You were not lucky enough (nor cursed, depending on your school of logic) to be BORN into being or wanting to be a Caregiver. That is unless of course you count being BORN into a family, or of a loved one, that now has a need for a Caregiver and the role is thrown at your feet. But that does not mean you are a BORN Caregiver... it means you were in the wrong (or right?) place at the wrong (or right?) time and you took on the responsibility.

When this happened, when your world changed was the day and time when you we reborn as a person and BORNE as a Caregiver b accepting that burden or responsibility.

It doesn't come naturally to you, but you find yourself in a position where you must learn to provide Care to a more vulnerable person. Thus, you are being or have been NURTURED (trained, developed, encouraged) to become a Caregiver... and to become one fast!

And because this is an obligation rather than a calling you take no intrinsic joy in doing it... it is purely an obligation, a duty, a responsibility.

So now your personal dilemma is that whenever you find yourself NOT answering the call of duty, not fulfilling your obligation or responsibility you are inviting guilt into your thought processes because you are, in essence, failing someone.

And in failing someone else, you are failing yourself and you have to choose between guilt and/or anger.

YOU MIGHT BE A **NURTURE** CAREGIVER *if...*
YOU FEEL GUILTY WHEN YOU TAKE CARE OF YOURSELF FIRST AND ANGRY WHEN YOU DON'T!

You will notice that nowhere in this book have I spoken of who, or how, we are Caring for whomever it is we are Caring for by whatever means.   That is intentional.   In this book the term Caregiver is far more about how a person feels about themselves and what and why they do certain things than it is about what they actually, physically do for Others.

I have purposefully not defined or described the Others that these Caregivers care for, whether they be a husband, spouse, child, patient, neighbor, parent, etc... nor the reason these people need care whether it be due to trauma, a congenital need, a physical or psychological need and so forth... nor where they Care for them whether it be at home, work, group, private, public... nor have I spoken on duration or frequency... live-in, institutional, long distance, community based, daily, 24/7, weekly etc...

You get the point. I am purposely avoiding the definition of a Caregiver by specifically how, what, where or to whom they provide Care... more directly, I am speaking about how they feel when they do what they do and why they do what they do!

This is more a spiritual, psychological and emotional definition than a physical or practical one.

And again, this is done on purpose.

I have had many a Caregiver take me to task for calling myself a

Caregiver... oh, they love that I am and call myself the "Defender Of Caregivers!" but they get upset at times when I call myself a Caregiver.

Why?

Well, in their mind, a Caregiver is someone who does what they do, how they do it, and for similar types of people in similar (or greater) degrees of effort... It is as though there is some imaginary Caregiver bar that we must each get over in order to be called a Caregiver.

They view it almost as if there is some diminishing value to the term Caregiver where, if it is used in the wrong setting or circumstance, it loses meaning or value. As if it were an insult to the other Caregivers who are using the term and providing services at the "proper" level!

What is the proper level?

How is the level determined and who determines it?

Whatever the answer, where does this judgment end?

If we all carry our burdens and responsibilities differently, how are we to determine who qualifies as a Caregiver and who does not? How do we know who gets to wear the Caregiver button?

Regardless of how you become or became a Caregiver...here you are!

Whether by Nature or by Nurture, you are a Caregiver, you frequently find yourself deferring your own needs to meet the needs of Others. And, as a Nurture Caregiver, this is a learned, not a Natural behavior. That in itself, learning to be something you Naturally are not, is inherently stressful.

When you are being forced by circumstance to change how you act, and to focus on the needs of Others more than your own needs; you are essentially being required to neglect yourself.

The subtle message is that anytime you concentrate on yourself it is at the expense of Others and leads not only to frustration when you don't or can't do it but to guilt when you do!

Unlike the Nature Caregiver who derives some pleasure through pleasing Others for you, the Nurture Caregiver, you take no pleasure and view it as a burden... essentially, you have the double whammy of being expected to take care of Others first and the inability to feel good about what you are doing because at some level you may resent it!

In fact, instead of being proud of it, you feel guilty about it!

This is allowing your feelings to be overwhelmed by circumstance; it is a passive act. You are allowing the circumstances to dictate your mood.

You are dabbling in EMOTIONAL REASONING (Caregiver Distortion #7) where you believe, "I feel it therefore it must be true!" In this way you are connecting your feelings, your emotions, with your self-worth or value.

In these moments you are failing to HONOR yourself (and your efforts) as you Care for Others!

You experience resentment THEREFORE you feel guilt. You are connecting the two as if it is real and valid.

It is not!

I call this the ERGO effect... Experience Resentment, Guilt Overload!

Let's visit the dictionary once again...

ergo
-sentence connector
1. therefore, hence

You experience resentment ERGO (therefore, hence) you feel guilt.

Sound familiar?

So how does the Nurture Caregiver turn this around?

They own it, they embrace it, they expect it... they HONOR themselves as they Care for Others... they choose their own attitude and here is how they do it!

The Nurture Caregiver must take charge of their own emotions by EXPECTING and EMBRACING what is a natural and expected reaction for them... yes, they should EXPECT and EMBRACE resentment for the role they are being required to play!

If they EXPECT and EMBRACE resentment rather than

EXPERIENCE resentment they can ACCEPT it as Natural and expected rather than be subjected to viewing it as a character flaw or weakness via distorted emotional reasoning.

If a certain feeling is EXPECTED and you can EMBRACE it what is there to feel guilty about?

The dynamic of EXPECTING and EMBRACING resentment changes the dynamic to this...

ERGO becomes: Embrace Resentment, Guilt is Obliterated.

If you go to work every day (perhaps for decades) to a job you don't necessarily enjoy out of a sense of responsibility do you feel guilty about it?

No!

You may resent it, but you don't feel guilty about it.

Because you Expect, Anticipate and Embrace your resentment you are able to see the value in your sacrifice!

You can even take some quiet pride in providing for your family even while doing something you do not love... you HONOR yourself while you work for Others!

Much of what DOC is trying to do for the Nurture Caregiver is to teach them through increased Awareness to not only Accept these feelings as Natural and unavoidable but to Anticipate, Embrace and Expect them... in doing so the Nurture Caregiver can choose their response rationally rather than emotionally.

You might be a nurture Caregiver *if...* you EMBRACE your emotions ERGO you can HONOR yourself (and your efforts) as you care for Others!

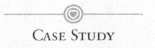

Case Study

*The case studies used in this book are real; and represent
Caregivers that are active members of the "Defender of Caregivers!" Fan Club.
Names have been changed as a courtesy to these amazing people.*

The Reluctant Caregiver (NURTURE Caregiver)

The dirty little secret behind the NURTURE Caregiver is that,
well, these are not necessarily NURTURing people. The term
NURTURE Caregiver is primarily referencing the "Learning"
aspect of the NATURE vs. NURTURE debate. These Caregivers
have Learned this behavior due to the necessity that they ACT
like a Caregiver; they have no choice but to defer their own needs
and satisfy the needs of Others.

This story is about a man... a Male Caregiver (that is purely
coincidental and is not meant to imply that women are
NATURAL Caregivers and Men are Reluctant Caregivers that
must be forced into the role) who I have known for years because
he is a dear friend. We will call him Steve. While I was running
Hospitals and Nursing Homes, I watched him take care of, Love,
fight, resent and cherish his mother.

He was devoted to her but he was not naturally or classically
a Loving Caregiver in a traditional way. Steve took great care
of his mom and put together a network of friends and semi-
professional Caregivers around the clock. He took care of all the
financial responsibilities and even made sure his mom was part
of family events and vacations. Because he was often stressed
or conflicted in his schedules, he sometimes resented these
responsibilities and intrusions on his life (but he would never say
so; which is also a part of this Dilemma... it is not appropriate to
outwardly complain).

Steve took care of everything thoroughly and diligently.
During a brief stint following his mother's surgery, he told the
nursing home, "I assure you, my mother is both destitute AND

homeless!" because together they had planned and implemented the plan of her estate with painstaking detail.

Later, Steve would commit to build an addition on his home with the plans of having his mother move in and live with him and his young family. This was done with trepidation because frankly, neither he nor his mother really wanted it to come to this; she didn't want to intrude and, well, he was glad to defer to her wishes on that subject (that was well-handled).

Ultimately, his mom was hit with an unforeseen illness that took her earlier than either of them had expected. She never did get to live in that beautiful addition. Steve was left feeling guilt instead of pride; he faulted himself for not doing more, sooner or better. "I could have built that addition sooner.... I should have eliminated the fireplace (but she did want it) and finished the room sooner." I should have done it! (SHOULD STATEMENT – Caregiver Distortion #8)

Finally, in addition to remorse for having lost his mother he was also filled with regret from his role as a Caregiver because felt he "failed" her when all who knew him held him in AWE for his dedication. He did not see any of this in himself and took no satisfaction from being a Caregiver.

DOC Comments...

Steve is a personal friend and I witnessed this relationship unfold for close to 10 years. His relationship with his mother was amazing! Frustrating? Yes, but amazing. His mom was demanding but not incessantly so; He was devoted but not incessantly so... he did what needed to be done but did not obsess over it... she made demands and had expectations, but was practical in the end. He expressed his guilt on several occasions, but did not seem to overcompensate and act out of guilt.

For the most part, he was in balance and did not delve into Distorted Thinking with the exception of one thing... he did not take credit for what he did for his mother and he allowed his unrealistic guilt to affect his opinion of himself. .... He often dabbled in SHOULD STATEMENTS (Caregiver Distortion #8) where he would declare one if his many perceived failures and suggest to himself that he SHOULD do better or more. Should Statements are a distortion! They do not serve as self motivation, they are self-mutilation; even if you do the things you SHOULD do you take no satisfaction because you have already declared that you SHOULD do them anyway! There is no win in doing or not-doing something you believe you SHOULD do!

His "therapy" and awareness came after his mother died... I applied the principles of the DOC's L.A.W. in our many conversations. This was a role reversal of sorts as Steve had supported me years earlier when I went through my divorce and some career challenges... he always told me "It is what it is!" As I Listened intently to him and then Advised him honestly and Worked with him to realize that what he did for his mother was amazing and rare... very few families actually pull it off and allow aging in place as successfully as he did... he was stubborn and held onto his unfounded but profoundly felt guilt for a long time.

After a while, I and others slowly began to win the battle. I told him, "It is what it is!" Eventually, his guilt faded and I believe he grew to be proud of his devotion to her...

He fought the L.A.W. but the L.A.W. won!

CHAPTER 4

The World According to DOC!

The CAREGIVER in YOU!

No matter what type of Caregiver you are - or aren't - to those among us that are not yet convinced there is a Caregiver in you, you must know this... you are flawed as a HUMAN BEING! LOL... yep, I said it... you are a FLAWED HUMAN BEING! After all, you ARE a HUMAN BEING so by definition you are FLAWED! But get this... you are perfectly flawed!

My good friend, fellow speaker, and spiritual adviser, Naval Commander Drew Brown (son of "Bundini" Brown, corner man and spiritual advisor to three-time heavy weight champion of the world and self-proclaimed, "Greatest of All Time" Muhammad Ali) always reminds me... "Lonny," he says, "your life is perfect! You just don't know it yet!"   Thank you Drew... (to learn more about Drew visit him at www.DrewBrown.net)

So, if DOC could be so bold as to call himself a "spiritual advisor" he would remind all of his Caregiver disciples that "you are a flawed human being...you may not know it yet but you are perfectly flawed for the role of Caregiver!"

The very things that perhaps make you flawed and vulnerable to the Chronic Episodic Depression scenario of the Caregiver's Dilemma are also the very things that make you a perfect Caregiver!

But you must also remember that perfection is also a flaw. Hey, I have already written this before. Let's jump to another BLOG from the www.DefenderOfCaregivers.com website:

WHY PERFECTION LEADS TO DEFECTION!

(Cognitive Distortion #1: "All-or-Nothing Thinking!)

There are tons of management books that talk about moving individuals, teams and organizations on a path toward constant improvement.

For people in Healthcare, some decisions ARE life and death.

There often needs to be a zero-tolerance objective; but this cannot be allowed to spill over into management of people, or of people managing themselves. It's fine for tasks, procedures, projects; not for people or relationships.

If you lead from a perspective and expectation of Perfection, people will ultimately show you Defection… they will not be lead into a fantasy world they know does not exist!

Defection is the only logical choice! If not Defection a forced pursuit of Perfection leads to anxiety and depression and I didn't want to write an article entitled, "Why Perfection Leads to Depression!" when there is a better choice: Defection!

Expecting perfection of your people (or yourself) is an invitation for them to leave because that is the only way they can meet your expectations.

Let me put it another way: as a singer (which I am not), the only perfect note I can hit is silence. If I want to be perfect or even good, I will never be able to sing!

But if I want to enjoy myself, express myself and project myself into life's chorus, if I want to participate and join the team, I and those around me must accept that I can't hit the high notes, or sometimes even the low notes. I, we, must accept less than perfection, or I cannot participate.

What we should demand and expect is enthusiastic participation; a genuine desire to achieve a common goal.

If your intentions are noble and efforts sincere, if you are doing something good; good enough is good enough!

We get away with nothing in life; everything we do comes back to us...

It is necessary to commit a perfect crime; but a flawed act of kindness is, well, good enough. If you are trying to take from someone or something you better wait to be Perfect in your execution; if you are trying to give to someone "good enough" now is much better then Perfect later or not at all... just do it! Good enough is good enough!

Asking for perfection of others is like telling them you don't like the way they are NOW; expecting perfection of yourself is the same thing! You don't like the way YOU are now!

The need for perfection is a cognitive distortion known as "All-or-Nothing Thinking" (Cognitive Distortion #1) where you see things in black and white. If your performance falls short of perfect, you see yourself as a total failure.

Finally... we have found perfection... as a total failure! A perfect failure! Wow! How easy was that?

Seeking perfection is itself a form of Defection. You are rejecting reality and attempting to Defect from it; the world is not Perfect in isolation, it is Perfect because of its Defects and that we accept it; we choose to participate in it, to enjoy it!

Caregivers choose to serve others with genuine enthusiasm and a desire to achieve a common goal!

I have often said that Caregivers are Perfectly Flawed... their personality dictates that they take their satisfaction through pleasing others rather than themselves.

So, in effect, they have a Defect in their ego; they need to please others in order to achieve satisfaction for themselves... thus, they possess the Perfect Defect for a successful career in healthcare.

Perfection is not only a fantasy, it is not even desirable. If you, or the situation you are in is Perfect; why would it ever change? It would/could never evolve; it would become routine, mundane, dare I say average.

Here we have demonstrated that Perfection is a Defect in and of itself and therefore there can be no such thing as Perfect.

*If you ask people (yourself) to pursue something they (you)
cannot possibly obtain, you are inviting them (yourself) to
withdraw, to Defect, from the journey.*

*I always ask; "when you are running on the treadmill of life
do you know if you are Seeking Success or running From
Failure? (an original Quote from: "Get Out of Bed and Go
to Work!" and "A.W.E.S.O.M.E Living!" Keynote/Plenary
addresses)*

*If you have issues, personal or professional, you are aware of
them and you embrace, celebrate, accommodate and achieve
things by navigating around them, your life is already Perfect.
You just don't know it yet. You are Perfectly flawed... you are
a Caregiver!*

THE PERFECTLY FLAWED – VIRTUAL CAREGIVER

Let's talk about a Perfect Flaw in this book. Something you may
have noticed by now... we have not once spoken about the people
or persons all these different Caregivers are Caring for... what type
of Care they need and how much or for how long... we haven't even
spoken about where they are being cared for or whether it is temporary or permanent, occasional or around the clock... and to the
casual reader that might be a FLAW. But guess what, I view it as a
Perfect Flaw because none of that matters!

Whether you are a follower of Popeye's world or that of Aristotle or,
frankly, if you don't accept either version, still you remain here and
you keep reading for a reason... so let us assume this...

YOU MIGHT BE A CAREGIVER *if...*
YOU HAVE REACHED CHAPTER 5 AND PAGE 49
OF THIS BOOK AND YOU ARE STILL READING IT

If you don't believe Popeye nor Aristotle, if you wish to ignore all of this up to this point then let me ask you a question: Why are you a Caregiver?

Because we already determined that you are indeed a Caregiver. By what virtue did you become a Caregiver? Why are you here?

You might be a Caregiver (by Virtue) *if...*
YOU FIND YOURSELF HERE AND CARING FOR OTHERS BUT YOU DON'T KNOW WHY

You are saying to yourself, "I am definitely not a NATURAL Caregiver... I hate that I am caught in the middle of it; I take no pleasure from it; in fact, I resent it; and I am not upset that I resent it; I am upset because I resent it! I don't feel guilty like a NURTURE Caregiver is supposed to feel... I am angry! I am doing something I don't want to be doing and I refuse to accept that I have somehow adopted a Caregiver Personality along the way!"

Ok then, why are you doing it? "Because I have no choice," you say, "Someone had to do it!" Well, yes, someone did have to do it, but it didn't have to be you! You are doing it because it is the virtuous thing to do and you are a man or woman of virtue.

Dictionary.com describes virtue as:
Vir·tue
—noun
1. moral excellence; goodness; righteousness.
2. conformity of one's life and conduct to moral and ethical principles; uprightness; rectitude.
—idioms
3. by / in virtue of, by reason of; because of: to act by virtue of one's legitimate authority.
4. make a virtue of necessity, to make the best of a difficult or unsatisfactory situation.

Somewhere, somehow...out of morality, goodness, righteousness, conformity and by reason of necessity...You are a *virtual* Caregiver!

Vir·tu·al
—adjective
5. being such in power, force, or effect, though not actually or expressly such.

As a virtual Caregiver you are in power, force or effect, though you are not actually or expressly a Caregiver! I have pretty much painted you into a corner. Sorry! Now deal with it and I mean that your anger may not be inward (yet) but because it has no safe place to go that is where it will turn and you will find yourself smack in the middle of the Caregiver's Dilemma just as much as any other true NATURAL or NURTURE Caregiver, but I guess yours will be a virtual Dilemma?

Either way the answer to the Dilemma is the same for all types of Caregivers. Caregivers by NATURE (BORN), Caregivers by NURTURE (BORNE) and Virtual Caregivers, too!

The bottom line is this. Being a Caregiver is like sleeping with the enemy. It represents constant (yet not always obvious) stress and when we are stressed we often suffer from distorted thinking.

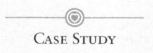

CASE STUDY

*The case studies used in this book are real; and represent
Caregivers that are active members of the "Defender of Caregivers!" Fan Club.
Names have been changed as a courtesy to these amazing people.*

THE OBTUSE CAREGIVER (VIRTUAL CAREGIVER)

The Virtual Caregiver may actually be a NATURE or a
NURTURE Caregiver; it is too soon to tell. In the case of the
Virtual Caregiver they likely have very strong Caregiver traits in
certain aspects of their lives but their routines and relationships
are mature and developed and decidedly do not revolve around
the need or desire to be a Caregiver. The Virtual Caregiver is
likely to be an outgoing type who over commits and is involved
with civic functions, and travels in well established social and
professional circles.

In this Case Study our Virtual Caregiver is a man, his duties,
responsibilities and relationships are well established; perhaps
OVER-ESTABLISHED. He is busy with his career, his family,
and his own personal pursuits. He is protective of his time
and is slow to commit to schedules because of an innate
subconscious feeling that he is already stretched too thin.

While he is committed to his family and truly loves being with
them he is very aware that lately, these activities (holidays,
special events) seem to take more and more energy out of
him; he even notices that the energy drain seems more in the
planning and preparation than in the actual execution of and
participation in the events.

His mother, who he deeply respects, appreciates and admires,
is increasingly demanding things of him. Small things; in fact,
really small things...so small in fact that he sees no value in
doing them, but nonetheless feels obligated, even pressured, into
doing them. And in doing them he takes no joy or satisfaction

despite the overt show of appreciation he receives for having done them. He realizes that this dynamic is nonsensical and is based on his value system and not his mother's; yet because he does not value what he has done for her, because he values the time he spent doing the task more so than the benefit of having the task done he feels anxious and frustrated. Instead he envisions all the valuable things he COULD and SHOULD do for her instead of wasting his time on these smaller non-value-added services. He is torn. On one hand he wishes he could do more, even searches ways to do more, but does not value or appreciate the things he actually does. This causes him guilt, worry, and occasional insomnia.

This man, the Virtual Caregiver, is not even aware he is already in a Caregiving relationship and, because of that, he is not reaping the intrinsic rewards and benefits of receiving satisfaction through pleasing others that a NATURAL Caregiver might obtain; nor does he get to give himself any of the credit that might be due the NURTURE Caregiver for doing something they view as "benevolent" this is all work and no joy, all guilt and no satisfaction. He is angry at the world because of the way he feels. The Virtual Caregiver is squarely in a full-blown Caregiver's Dilemma before he or she even knows he is a Caregiver.

His relief came from an epiphany like of experience that allowed him to become AWARE of the role he was playing and the relationship he was in; that it was partially NATURAL and partially learned (NURTURE-based) ... and he ACCEPTED his role as...the "Defender Of Caregivers!"

That's right...the Virtual Caregiver is ME/DOC!

Thank you for sharing my story, my journey and I welcome you into my own V.A.L.U.E. Circle known as the "Defender of Caregivers!"

DOC Comments...

I know that was a nice and dramatic end with a suspenseful build-up and a well-delivered, profound finish, but you still have to read the rest of the book!

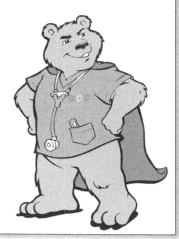

CHAPTER 5

Why Caregivers are Distorted and Contorted!

D aniel Batson, a Princeton-trained psychologist defines
EMPATHY as "a motivation oriented towards the other."

Yeah, pretty much the same definition, but a lot fewer words, that
Myers-Briggs provided to describe "the Caregiver!"

Dictionary.com provides this definition for EMPATHY.

Em·pa·thy

–noun

1. *the intellectual identification with or vicarious experiencing of
the feelings, thoughts, or attitudes of another.*

The hallmark of the Caregiver is EMPATHY… through the
vicarious experiencing of the feelings, thoughts, or attitudes of
others; and by being motivated towards others… they are essentially
living more than one life… they live their own life and that of those
they care for!

Let us now look at depression. There are two types of depression;
episodic and chronic. A thorough discussion of depression is well
beyond the scope of this book (and remember, DOC is not a doctor
or trained therapist) so we will use the following quick, easy and
non-clinical definitions for the purposes of this book:

Depression: a disorder of guilt, sadness, hopelessness and passivity; the common cold of mental illnesses.

Episodic Depression: lasts less than two years, has a clear beginning.

Chronic Depression: lasts more than two years without a two-month break; the clear beginning is not discernable or memorable.

DOC holds that Caregivers, by virtue of their EMPATHIC ways are subjected to a type of chronic stress that results from essentially living more than one life. They not only experience their own life and circumstances they truly FEEL (empathy) the life and circumstance of others.

The Caregiver can never get away from calamitous circumstances because it is in their nature to seek them. They are attracted like flies to the light toward people in need and as a result they go from one EPISODE of depressing circumstances to another to another and so on.

There is a scene in the comedic/dramatic play "Defending the Caregiver!" where the antagonist Lon Kieffer and the protagonist "DOC" are having a dialogue. DOC says, "Don't you realize that you are depressed? Don't you realize you need help?"

Lon says, "Yeah DOC, I am depressed! But I don't need help. You see…there are two kinds of depression. Chronic, where you need help; and episodic, where you just need time. I have Chronic Episodic Depression. I don't need help, I just need more time!"

DOC says, "OMG your condition is worse than I thought!"

You might be a Caregiver *if…*
YOU KNOW ENOUGH TO BE DANGEROUS, BUT NOT ENOUGH TO KNOW YOU ARE DANGEROUS (TO YOURSELF)

The Caregiver is lost in the game. Actually, they are not lost, they know where they are; but they have lost themselves. They have lost insight into what they need to take care of themselves.

In this way, the Caregiver can very likely suffer from what I affectionately call Chronic Episodic Depression and have no insight into the condition. They have lost themselves already but have not yet had the benefit of perspective or of walking past a proverbial mirror so as to notice it on a conscious level.

The Caregiver that has reached a breaking point or that suddenly is no longer engaged in the act and art of Caregiving may find themselves in a full blown depressive state (a loss of identity), then may realize that they have been in one for quite some time and never noticed it!

For these Caregivers, their depressive episodes have a clear beginning but never a clear end as they perhaps slipped unnoticed into the next new episode with its own clear beginning until it is all a blur and they are correct; it wasn't them feeling it to begin with... but it eventually becomes them!

For the Caregiver that is fully engaged in the act and process of providing Care for another, they may perhaps not notice the underlying feelings of guilt, sadness or hopelessness because they are prevented from wallowing in the final depressive symptom of passivity.

They are so active, so productive, so giving to and for another how could they possibly be suffering from depression? This is the true silent killer (with apologies to those with high blood pressure)!

THE DISTORTING FORCES OF STRESS

Dr. Burns, in his book "Feeling Good: The New Mood Therapy," shares with us his list of Cognitive Distortions (Appendix C).

These are thinking patterns that people utilize when under stress or when, for one reason or another, are not thinking clearly.

Dr. Burns is considered the godfather of Mood Therapy and in his book "Feeling Good" he describes how to combat feelings of depression so you can develop greater self-esteem. This best-selling book has sold more than 4 million copies worldwide. In a national survey of mental health professionals, "Feeling Good" was rated number one, out of a list of 1,000 books, as the most frequently recommended self-help book on depression in the United States.

I know, because my own personal doctor recommended it to me

several years ago. (NOTE: DOC and Lon are not smart enough to think of all of this themselves. Just know that you are NOT alone in this journey it's just that some of us speak and write books... HINT, wink, nod!)

Once I learned personally, and became aware of the phenomenon of how chronic stress had contorted my own way of seeing the world (my chronic-episodic view), I began to make some very profound observations.

I began to observe that those same Caregivers I referenced earlier, the ones that exhibited an almost shared (and later clinically confirmed by Myers-Briggs) personality were also exhibiting many of these Cognitive Distortions. And so, the logic being that Cognitive Distortions are exhibited by people under stress and that Caregivers are chronically under stress... perhaps Chronically Distorted?

Remember that Elephant? Well, let's invite him back into the room, for there is no empirical evidence that this is true and Dr. Burns is silent on the issue of how his Cognitive Distortions become Caregiver Distortions in the humble and anecdotal opinion of DOC the "Defender of Caregivers!"

Okay, now that I magically made an Elephant appear...POOF... gone again!

Throughout this book, I have made the occasional reference to these "Caregiver Distortions" and I doubt you objected much to them... and I assure you, I don't share this opinion that Caregivers are chronically prone to distorted thinking lightly; it is a carefully considered opinion yet lacking in the true pedigree in psychiatry, psychology, etc. to make it fact. Once again, it is intuitively and philosophically true that...

> IF those under stress are prone to suffer from
> Cognitive Distortions (negative thinking patterns)
> AND if Caregivers are under chronic stress
> THEN Caregivers are Chronically prone to suffer
> from Cognitive Distortions.

Now, I had a major interest (but not a minor degree) in Philosophy while in college, so that is good enough for me. The result is... drum roll please...the following:

YOU MIGHT BE A CAREGIVER *if...*
YOU FIND YOURSELF SOMETIMES THINKING IN EXTREMES ONLY TO LOOK BACK ON EVENTS OR DECISIONS AS BEING LESS CRITICAL THAN YOU ORIGINALLY THOUGHT!

~~~~~~~~

YOU MIGHT BE A CAREGIVER *if...*
YOU RECOGNIZE AND RESEMBLE SOME OF THESE EXAMPLES OF CAREGIVER DISTORTIONS

We all (not just Caregivers) tend to think in extremes and when traumatic events happen, we think that way even more. These are common cognitive distortions (they become Caregiver Distortions only because the life and empathic nature of a Caregiver chronically subjects them to traumatic events; this is in the opinion of DOC).

Take a look and see if any of them are getting in your way.

1. *All-or-nothing thinking:* You see things in black and white categories. If your performance falls short of perfect, you see yourself as a total failure.

2. *Overgeneralization:* You see a single negative event as a never-ending pattern of defeat.

3. *Mental filter:* You pick out a single negative detail and dwell on it exclusively so that your vision of all reality becomes darkened, like the drop of ink that discolors the entire glass of water.

4. *Disqualifying the positive:* You reject positive experiences by insisting they "don't count" for some reason or other. You maintain a negative belief that is contradicted by your everyday experiences.

5. *Jumping to conclusions:* You make a negative interpretation, even though there are no definite facts that convincingly support your conclusion.

a. Mind reading: You arbitrarily conclude that someone is reacting negatively to you and don't bother to check it out.

b. The Fortune teller error: You anticipate that things will turn out badly and feel convinced that your prediction is an already-established fact.

6. *Magnification (catastrophizing) or minimization:* You exaggerate the importance of things (such as your goof-up or someone else's achievement) or you inappropriately shrink things until they appear tiny (your own desirable qualities or the other fellow's imperfections). This is also called the "binocular trick."

7. *Emotional reasoning:* You assume that your negative emotions necessarily reflect the way things really are: "I feel it, therefore it must be true."

8. *Should statements:* You try to motivate yourself with shoulds and shouldn'ts, as if you had to be whipped and punished before you could be expected to do anything. "Musts" and "oughts" are also offenders. The emotional consequence is guilt. When you direct should statements toward others, you feel anger, frustration, and resentment.

9. *Labeling and mislabeling:* This is an extreme form of overgeneralization. Instead of describing your error, you attach a negative label to yourself: "I'm a loser." When someone else's behavior rubs you the wrong way, you attach a negative label to him, "He's a damn louse." Mislabeling involves describing an event with language that is highly colored and emotionally loaded.

10. *Personalization:* You see yourself as the cause of some negative external event for which, in fact, you were not primarily responsible.

From: Burns, David D., MD. 1989. The Feeling Good Handbook. New York: William Morrow and Company, Inc.

BOOM, there it is! Or I should say, there they are!

The entire point behind this book, "You might be a Caregiver if..." is that I wanted you to know that!

I believe strongly everything about the Myers-Briggs version of

Caregiver; Popeye's opinions are equally valid and undeniable; Aristotle...come on, am I going to argue with Aristotle? Not...! But this, this is the mesh... these Caregiver Distortions are what I wanted to get to!

You see... at the core of all of this I believe that AWARENESS and ACCEPTANCE of who and why we are... Caregivers... can give us enough pause, enough confidence, enough clarity that we can help ourselves avoid thinking in distorted ways!

And this alone can break the cycle of the Caregiver's Dilemma and change the S.C.R.I.P.T. to allow the Caregiver to accept help and relieve themselves the burden of harshly judging themselves, eliminate guilt and unrealistic expectations... allow them to accept that..."it is what it is!"

I believe that the simple reminder that, and acknowledgment of, our naturally prone personality lending itself to these Caregiver Distortions can help us to combat this negative (distorted) way of thinking.

It can be the sort of... "yeah, I do that... I am so dumb!" epiphany type of awareness a good humorist offers to people as he mimics them accurately and amusingly if not lovingly.

Recognize yourself accurately and acutely in any given moment and you have a better shot of avoiding your destiny of negative outcomes of guilt, anger, anxiety and despair that come from Cognitive (Caregiver) Distortions and other Stinkin' Thinkin' processes.

We now have two ways of protecting our own precious little Caregiver hearts:

We become AWARE and ACCEPT
what, why and who we are...
We ACKNOWLEDGE
our tendency to think in distorted ways.

Wow, turns out we are insured by AAA!
(or is it just Triple-A? I am excited!)

Just think of Awareness, Acceptance and Acknowledgment as the Caregivers emotional roadside assistance as you travel on your life's journey!

And it doesn't hurt to have clear vision as you drive through life. Remember the Schnellen Eye-chart we showed you with the Caregiver at the center of the universe thinking that, "I am not happy unless you are happy!"?

Now that you have Triple-A protection you can also have 20/20 vision and see the world more clearly… you can learn to see the world with you still at the center of the universe but unaffected by the emotional whims of others;

DOC PROVIDES A CLEAR FUTURE VISION

In this new, clear view of the Universe, the Caregiver can still be immersed in the center of the world/universe but does not have to feel sorry (or responsible; PERSONALIZATION, Caregiver Distortion #10) simply because others are not happy. They are able to feel and be independent of Others!

You Can Go...

To:
A Caregivers view of the Universe when being properly DEFENDed by AWARENESS and ACCEPTANCE of the Caregivers Dilemma.

From:
A Caregiver's Distorted View of the Universe.

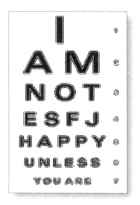

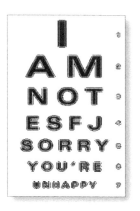

Why Caregivers are Contorted

Caregivers whether by NATURE, NURTURE or VIRTUE are either willingly or reluctantly in a position to do for others before they do for themselves.

Remember this passage from the Myers-Briggs "A Portrait of the Caregiver!"? -- You are extremely good at reading others, and often change your own manner to be more pleasing to whoever you're with at the moment. Yes, it's true, you will CONTORT yourself into the version of yourself that is most pleasing to Others.

The Caregiver, in essence, will "bend over backwards" to help others and they feel they MUST or at least SHOULD (SHOULD STATEMENTS, Caregiver Distortion #8) do this because it is expected of them by others or by themselves.

The Caregiver will always focus on what they SHOULD do rather than celebrate what they already DID! This can be fatalistic and self defeating characteristic... the Caregiver needs encouragement to focus on what they have already accomplished for one very simple reason:

> "The Caregiver must learn to take pride in what
> they have already DONE; because the
> Caregivers work never is DONE!"

How Caregivers Can Lose Themselves

Here are some of the ways a Caregiver can lose themselves while caring for Others.

If the Caregiver denies themselves the conscious acknowledgment of praise or a feeling of accomplishment until the work is done, they will never receive such praise because their work well never be done!

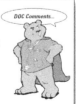

DOC Comments...

- *They do a great job and balance their responsibilities with apparent ease!*

- *They lose themselves because eventually they identify with what they do; they become their work. When people tell them they "are doing a great job!" they become the person that others admire and cease to be ordinary. The do not pursue singular or intrinsic joys or accomplishments.*

- *They do a great job and "cure" the person they are providing Care for.*

- *Yes, they have done a great thing, but they have lost their purpose, a piece of their identity, a source of pleasure is lost to them. They do not feel the sense of joy for a "job well done," they do not experience a relief; they experience a loss. It is like the gambler who finally wins big yet continues to gamble until he loses it all and finds that the winning was not as satisfying as the process of trying to win. The process is the prize, not the winning!*

- *They do a great job and serve nobly yet they "lose" the person they were Caring for.*

This is a double whammy, they do not take satisfaction out of the service they provided because they need to be actively involved in serving others to derive satisfaction from it; the sense of joy is dulled by the sense of loss. This represents a loss of both a loved individual and of a cherished role. The intellectual inevitability of this loss is no safeguard against the complete surprise emotionally for the Caregiver.

The bottom line to every one of the scenarios is hidden in an essay by Lon Kieffer entitled; "How to become a truly A.W.E.S.O.M.E. Human Being!" (and yes... H.U.M.A.N. is an Acronym). Read this excerpt where Lon discusses the "U" in H.U.M.A.N and the inherent need for Caregivers to:

Understand Success (and define: CARE) How do we define success in Healthcare (a Caregiving relationship)?

Dictionary.com defines CARE for others as: serious attention and protection. We must all learn that CARE is a model of independence NOT dependence. Our role is one of support, concern and protection, NOT doing things for others that they can do for themselves.   Caregiver at best is a temporary relationship where success and failure both define the end of the relationship. We must Understand (be AWARE of) and Accept things as they actually are; (either way, through success or by failure the Caregiving relationship will end) the trick is to know the difference!

The Caregivers G.O.D. Complex

Without this Understanding of what Care truly means the Caregiver is left reading from their S.C.R.I.P.T. and stuck in the quickening spin of the Caregiver's Dilemma... they will develop a G.O.D. complex.

The Caregiver expects great, even impossible things of themselves. They can NEVER do enough because they have no sense of how much is enough... as we said before... their work is never done and because they have either a desire to do more (Nature Caregiver) or a sense of obligation or commitment to do more (Nurture Caregiver) they begin to think of themselves with G.O.D.-like expectations.

But alas, they are not omnipotent... they have limits. They are not G.O.D. and when they finally realize this, they experience Guilt... when you start with Guilt and add to it continued and ever-increasing Obligation you frequently get Depression.

Guilt + Obligation = Depression

If DOC can help the Caregiver let go of their Guilt... and without the G in Guilt there can be no... (even DOC isn't going to finish that sentence!) well, without Guilt... the equation no longer equals Depression; it remains simply Obligation.

CHAPTER 6

How ACRONYMS and ANTAGONYMS can H.E.L.P. Caregivers!

OK...I started my career as a public figure as a humor-based motivational speaker (and I still do quite a lot of it...www. LonKieffer.com) and speakers love ACRONYMS.

So, I just had to put a few ACRONYMS in this book!

As you know an ACRONYM is a "word formed from the initial letters of a phrase or series of words."

EXAMPLE: TEAM   T - together

                         E - everyone

                         A - achieves

                         M - more

Also, as you know, ACRONYMS can be A.N.N.O.Y.I.N.G! Sometimes speakers rely on ACRONYMS too much and it becomes tedious...TRUST me.

TRUST   T - teamwork

             R - respect

             U - I got nothing, you?

             S - Sasquatch; does he really exist?

             T - terrific example of a BAD Acronym

So, with apologies I freely admit this next section could easily be called Acronym Alley! I hope it doesn't become too tedious. To break things up I will also introduce something called an Antagonym which is a word that can have two simultaneous meanings that are exactly opposite each other. The intent is to leave behind some recognizable and easily remembered words (Acronyms) that are inspirational and meaningful as words and as the deeper meaning of their definitions.

We will be using words, no Acronyms, like: H.O.P.E., V.A.L.U.E., L.A.W. and even the perhaps too long but poignant S.C.R.I.P.T. to name a few.

Acronyms can re-write the Caregiver's S.C.R.I.P.T.

So, now that you have read 67 or so pages telling how and why you're destined to chronically suffer from the Caregiver's Dilemma you're ready to curl up with a pillow and feel sorry for yourself, right? And to think, before you heard of DOC you didn't know how bad you had it right?

You were just cruising along doing what you do (Born Caregiver) or doing what you had to do (Borne Caregiver) and not thinking that you were destined to a life of chronic stress, guilt and possible depression. Boy, I bet you are glad you bought this book! Right? I HOPE not! Because that is NOT the picture I am trying to paint at all.

I have been accused by some Caregivers of "thinking Caregivers are these weak vulnerable people that need help and support just to function!" Because I describe Caregivers as, "emotional cripples always on the verge of a meltdown!" Quite the contrary! I believe Caregivers are the strongest, most able individuals in society.

When many are taking a free ride in the wagon, it is the Caregivers that are out front pulling and carrying the load; and that is the analogy I would like to stick with – Caregivers carrying a load, a burden.

Whether Born or BORNE it is still burdensome to Care for Others! And Caregivers are world-class in what they do! Imagine if you were a world-class weightlifter and you came into my gym for a competition. Wouldn't I be irresponsible if I allowed you to lift weights without a proper warm up; without a safety belt to protect your back; without a spotter in case you fall? That would be VERY irresponsible! Come back to reality. You are not a world-class weight lifter. You are a Caregiver!

On a daily basis, you carry far more than your own weight, yet when you come into the gym (out into the world) no one offers you any safety equipment; no warm up; no spotter. Instead, they essentially walk up to you and say, "How much weight you have on that bar? Looks heavy…mind if I add a few more pounds?"

How many times have you, the Caregiver, had people that are not your responsibility offer to add weight to your burden?

   • "Since you are going to pick up those prescriptions anyway, can you get mine, too?"

   • "Hey since you are going to be home with (fill in the blank) today, do you mind if my daughter comes over after school?"

I am sure you can come up with even more examples! The key here is that you do what you do so naturally others begin to take it for granted; they don't realize the load you carry because you carry it so well.

And that brings me back to my original point. You carry these burdens so naturally often times YOU don't know you are carrying them! That's the problem! I don't think you are weak, I think you are strong! You are not frail…but you are vulnerable!

If you do not become consciously AWARE of and ACCEPT the Caregiver's Dilemma as real, you are destined to suffer from it! You are in denial!

Those of you that are screaming inside your heads (or inside your living room!) that you are VERY aware of the burden you carry; that you feel stressed out every day; that you don't need to be told you carry your burdens naturally and well because you are drowning as you tread water and feel the weight getting heavier every day. Guess what?

You are already there. You are displaying the symptoms of the Caregiver's Dilemma! Not because you are overloaded with responsibilities but because you feel locked in and hopeless. Not only are you overwhelmed but you feel you have or are failing when you most likely are actually doing an amazing job against an impossible task. Well, HOPE springs eternal!

HOPE SPRINGS ETERNAL

Hope springs eternal in the human breast;
Man never Is, but always To be blest:
The soul, uneasy and confin'd from home,
Rests and expatiates in a life to come.
~ Alexander Pope, An Essay on Man, Epistle I (1733)

Let's break this down line by line...

Hope springs eternal in the human breast;
As humans, we are driven by our dreams, our visions, our desires

Man never Is, but always To be blest;
We often overlook that we are blest... and believe that somehow, someday, we will be more blest than now...

The soul, uneasy and confin'd from home,
It is natural to be restless and want more and to feel confined by responsibility

Rests and expatiates in a life to come.
Ah, to rest and be free to move around (expatiate) someday in the future!

It means that no matter the circumstances, man will always hope for the best, think that better things will come down the road. We may not always act our best, but we have the potential to be better in the future. No matter how bad things have been, they can always get better.

These are the feelings of man (or at least of Alexander Pope) as far back as 1733. These are normal everyday feelings, a touch of despair but HOPEful for the future.

The Caregiver who fails to realize that what he or she is experiencing is normal and is to be expected for someone carrying such a burden will inexorably spiral downward and into the Caregiver's Dilemma as if they are just an actor on the world's stage reading from a SCRIPT; they will...

- **S**ee only the despair and not the HOPE.

- **C**ontinue to live and act in denial of their burdens.

- **R**efuse assistance or acknowledge that they need help.

- **I**nvite feelings of guilt and/or inadequacy to mount.

- **P**ersist in their unrealistic expectations (of self)

- **T**hink ever increasingly using Caregiver Distortions

I believe, and have built much of the "Defender of Caregivers!" philosophy on this belief, that this cycle can be forever broken with two simple and closely related acts: increased AWARENESS and ACCEPTANCE.

If the Caregiver, through increased AWARENESS can understand that what is happening to them is not only normal, it is to be expected; and if they can therefore ACCEPT their feelings of anger, guilt, fear and anxiety as normal rather than a symptom of failure or inadequacy. Well, the HOPE can Spring Eternal for them once again.

DOC realizes the idea that merely increasing AWARENESS and ACCEPTANCE in the perspective of Caregivers can be therapeutic and helpful might seem overly simplistic but he also FEELS it very strongly so it must be true...right?

Hopefully, you have learned that believing something is true simply because you FEEL it strongly is a Caregiver Distortion (#7 Emotional Reasoning), but DOC not only FEELS it is true, he knows it is true because he has literature and research on his side. The fact that feelings of GUILT lead to depression is just that – a fact.

This fact has been researched and written over and over again. Quite frankly, I cannot choose a singular (or even several) sources to offer without excluding literally hundreds of other equally good or better sources. And guilt is the Hallmark of the Caregiver's Dilemma

The Natural Caregiver who takes pleasure out of pleasing others finds it difficult to please themselves directly and leaving others out of the equation. They may even feel selfish by taking care of themselves first.

YOU MIGHT BE A CAREGIVER *if...*
YOU DON'T NEED TO BE TAUGHT HOW TO TAKE CARE OF YOURSELF
YOU NEED TO BE GIVEN PERMISSION!

The Nurture Caregiver feels guilty because they don't always take pleasure out of serving others; they feel an obligation and then feel guilty (or angry at themselves) for NOT Giving more freely, more willingly.

YOU MIGHT BE A CAREGIVER *if...*
YOU FEEL GUILTY WHEN YOU TAKE CARE OF YOURSELF AND ANGRY WHEN YOU DON'T!

The Natural Caregiver feels guilty because they take satisfaction out of pleasing others; the Nurture Caregiver feels guilty because they don't!

So, the idea behind the DOC philosophy that AWARENESS and ACCEPTANCE are the secret to breaking through and out of the S.C.R.I.P.T. of the Caregiver's Dilemma is this simple equation:

A.A.R.P

I know, you are asking, what does the American Association of Retired Persons have to do with the Caregiver's Dilemma? Well, nothing. In this case A.A.R.P. stands for: Awareness, Acceptance, and Reject Pessimism

See, the key to the Caregiver's Dilemma is why Caregivers reach the breaking point; what is the straw that breaks the camel's back? There is no doubt that stress, empathy, obligation and responsibility are a burden on the Caregiver, but the proverbial straw that breaks the camel's back is guilt!

And this guilt comes from pessimism. The Caregiver becomes pessimistic. Not about the fact that they have a huge burden to carry; not about whatever ailment or career choice has placed them into the role of Caregiver. The Caregiver becomes pessimistic because they doubt themselves!

The Nature Caregiver can never do enough, can never get enough satisfaction so they do more and more and get further and further into their own dilemma and they feel that they are failing. Failing for them is not only against their own expectations, it is against their nature!

The Nurture Caregiver can never do enough because they don't get satisfaction from it. Their motivation is to avoid pain and because pain still comes they are not doing enough! They feel guilty for not doing enough and exhausted from trying.

Either way, both the Nature and the Nurture Caregiver feels that they are failing when in reality they are doing far more, in most cases, than is reasonable to expect. And yet, they feel guilty.

They feel guilty for vastly different reasons, but they feel it just the same and after guilt becomes pessimism because they don't know any different.

They don't know that this is all to be expected and in some ways should even be embraced. It is a validation that they are either acting Naturally or they are responsibly acting in a Nurturing way; and feeling like they are feeling at times is to be expected.

You might be a Caregiver *if*...
you believe, like Bethany Hamilton the
Soul Surfer does, that
"I don't need easy, I just need possible!"

Whether it be because you were BORN by Nature into it or BORNE by obligation into it; you are doing something that is NOT easy, but it is possible! How do I know it is possible? Because you are doing it...YOU are a Caregiver!

And if through AWARENESS and ACCEPTANCE we can encourage you to REJECT PESSIMMISM we are creating an environment where human nature can become greater than the Caregivers Dilemma. We can allow the Caregiver to once again believe that: H.O.P.E. does indeed Spring Eternal.

Why H.O.P.E. Springs Eternal

The Caregiver in YOU can live with HOPE if you;

> HONOR (be aware of) yourself as you care for others!

> OPENLY accept who and why you are YOU!

> PRACTICE self-loving acts daily!
> (until practice makes perfect)

> ENGAGE other Caregivers in VALUE based relationships.

When BAD is GOOD!

The old adage; "it is better to give than to receive" is, frankly, the Caregiver's worst rally cry!" Due to the Nature of the Natural Caregiver and Necessity for the Nurture Caregiver, they are already predisposed out of desire (Nature) or demand (Nurture) to give so much.

When you add into this equation an age-old belief and value such as it is better to give than to receive you have a lose-lose scenario for the Caregiver because they are encouraged to do something that might not be in their own best interests!

You might argue this on the surface – it is better to give than to receive – and the Caregiver takes satisfaction from Giving to (pleasing) Others! Perfect, right? Not so fast!

Remember the Caregiver's Dilemma. The Caregiver does not consciously accept the joy or pleasure they should receive from Giving. In fact, at the conscious level they almost willfully reject it, feel guilty by it or further obligated because of it. Again, they cannot win! But, they don't have to suffer this lose-lose scenario if they simply become AWARE of and ACCEPT that this is their natural dilemma – the Caregiver's Dilemma!

I believe strongly that the simple act of AWARENESS and ACCEPTANCE can be the protective bands around the Caregiver's

Heart that we discussed in the very earliest pages of this book. Here is why. Have you ever gone to bed knowing that tomorrow was going to be a great day? You knew the weather was going to be perfect and you had plans to enjoy the weather doing things you love with people you love (I will leave it to you fill in the blanks regarding what things you love to do and who you love to do those things with) but do you know the feeling I am talking about?

For some of us, it might be as simple as a walk in the park or a boat ride; for others it might be as complex as a hot-air balloon and a bottle of Champagne or…

You might be a Caregiver *if…*
YOU THINK A PERFECT DAY IS JUST NESTING AROUND THE HOUSE AND COOKING A LARGE MEAL FOR YOUR FAMILY (AND HAVING THEM ALL TOGETHER FOR ONCE TO EAT IT!)

Let's agree that we will leave the complex "perfect day" alone and just concentrate on the simple joys of everyday living; at least for th purposes of this discussion. I don't want to deny you any hot-air balloon rides!

So, you are going to bed envisioning your "perfect day" tomorrow. You are having trouble sleeping because your mind is racing ahead to your "perfect day" (or, because you are exhausted from Caregiving and can't keep your eyes open) either way, when you finally fall asleep you have an anticipatory smile in your heart, in your head and on your face.

Then tomorrow comes and you have your "perfect day"! That's it. End of story. Nothing dramatic! So, how do you feel? Your day is now over, and it was the "perfect day"! How do you feel? Well, let me help you with this because I know exactly how this feels.

Your emotions are actually mixed. You had a great day and you fee it with every bone in your body and every piece of gray matter in your brain, but you also know it is over. It is now a memory instead of a vision and you are already wondering what is better, the vision or the memory?

There is nothing negative about this; it is natural for everyone. Not just Caregivers because, you see, memories fade where as visions grow! It is a reality for us all. The realities of things are rarely as powerful as our imagination of those same things!

Let us return to the Caregiver personality. The reality of what we do for others ALWAYS pales in comparison to our own imagination or vision of what we SHOULD (SHOULD STATEMENTS, Caregiver Distortion #8) or could have done for Others!

As Caregivers, it would be wonderful if we could become AWARE of and ACCEPT this reality. Then, when we disappoint ourselves for not doing more or better or even enough we can smile at how Natural this feeling is. We can celebrate this negative feeling as a validation of how wonderful (and how unrealistic) our vision we have of ourselves truly is. This might be one opportunity to make a negative a positive.

I feel bad about myself because I AM SO DAMN GOOD! That's right. BAD is GOOD! If you feel BAD it is because you are GOOD! So, wait for it...wait for it... "Girl... you BAD!"

Remember "back in the day" when FAT became good? The vernacular was, "that girl is so FAT!" (DOC is aware he is on a slippery slope here! Lon will let DOC take this one!) then we all learned that FAT was good because it was spelled PHAT as in, Pretty Hot And Tempting!

It was around that same time that BAD became GOOD (it is called an Antagonym [Appendix D] and yes, that is a real expression where a word can mean the opposite of itself) and as a Caregiver you had no idea they were talking about you did you? Well, now you know!

YOU MIGHT BE A CAREGIVER *if*...
YOU NOW KNOW THAT "YOU BAD" REALLY MEANS
"YOU ARE GOOD"...
AND YOU KNOW WHY YOU ARE SOOOO
DAMN BAD/GOOD!

(go 'head with your GOOD/BAD self girl!)

Why, you ask, did I pick such obscure a concept as an ANTAGONYM to make this point? Well, first, I would say, "Congratulations on using ANTAGONYM in a sentence" and then I would answer, "Because Caregivers often look at BAD as GOOD and GOOD as BAD!"

Let's refer back to some of the earliest pages of this book where we learned about the Caregiver Personality as defined by Myers-Briggs. Where the Caregiver gets pleasure by pleasing others.

We know from studying human behavior that there are generally two categories for motivation:

- Pain, that most of us move away from, want less of
- Pleasure, that most of us move towards, want more of

The Caregiver's Dilemma is that this is all distorted by the simple fact that their pain also provides them pleasure; they often cannot seek or receive one without also inviting the other along for the ride

The Nature Caregiver receives pleasure (satisfaction) through pain (providing for others); in order to get something GOOD they must do something BAD (or at least difficult).

The Nurture Caregiver must also seek pleasure (avoidance of pain) through pain (providing unnatural services) ; in order to avoid something BAD (guilt) they must do something GOOD (provide something to others).

This conundrum also blurs the lines of perception where two people can see the same thing and one perceive it as BAD the other as GOOD. So, you have the same things that are also opposites; ANTAGONYMS!

For the Caregiver it truly IS better to give than to receive for they receive pleasure through giving. So, for the Caregiver, GIVING ends up meaning GETTING! This is or can be both GOOD and BAD.

Technically, GIVING meaning GETTING may not be an ANTAGONYM because I can't provide an acceptable literary (literature) example of it such as:

cut (get into a line)

cut (get out of a class)

But I can provide an acceptable literal example:

give (meaning to give to others)

GIVE (meaning to GET satisfaction for a Caregiver!)

Oh, here is my acceptable literary example:

YOU MIGHT BE A CAREGIVER *if...*
FOR YOU IT LITERALLY IS BETTER TO GIVE
THAN IT IS TO RECEIVE!

I have seen it all over the course of my career. Caregivers who have given so much and for so long that when they are no longer needed, they find they have lost their identity, their purpose.

Caregivers create dependency. Create the need for their efforts and prevent the person they are caring for from becoming more independent.

So, in some ways when the person or things a Caregiver is caring for are doing GOOD it is subconsciously BAD for the Caregiver and when they are doing BAD it is subconsciously GOOD!

Some Caregivers are NOT stressed but fulfilled by their role, by the services they provide. But don't be fooled, these Caregivers are suffering from the Caregiver's Dilemma just as much as their fellow Caregivers are back in that deep water treading with lead weights strapped to them!

The problem is they don't know it and perhaps never will. Whereas the Caregiver that is treading water is afraid of drowning, the content Caregiver is afraid of walking! They would not know how to act if they lost their role as a Caregiver. The drowning Caregiver is afraid of losing themselves; the swimming Caregiver is afraid of finding themselves! Either way, they... or...

YOU MIGHT BE A CAREGIVER *if...*
YOU GIVE YOURSELF TO OTHERS
THEN WONDER WHAT HAPPENED TO YOU!

Either way, the Caregiver relationship will eventually end one day and the Nature Caregiver may feel a loss of purpose (self) and the Nurture Caregiver may feel a loss of opportunity for having not been able to express themselves fully while Caregiving.

V.A.L.U.E. Circles: Giving and Receiving

Once the Caregiver has a heightened Awareness and Acceptance of who, what and why they are unique and perfectly flawed for their challenges, they can begin to have and seek relationships based on V.A.L.U.E. that can help them change their own behavior.

Changing the Caregiver's behavior and beliefs is the key!

In his book "Change or Die: The Three Keys to Change at Work and in Life" Alan Deutschman talks about why programs like Alcoholics Anonymous and Weight Watchers work when it comes to changing people's behavior.

He says it is because they have catchy memorable two-word, same letter titles. Apparently if we have any hope of success we should be known as the Caregivers Coalition, rather than the "Defender Of Caregivers!" – just kidding!

What if you were given that choice? Change or Die! We're talking actual life and death now; your own life and death. What if a well-informed, trusted authority figure said you had to make difficult and enduring changes in the way you think, feel, and act? If you didn't, your time would end soon—a lot sooner than it had to. Could you change when change mattered most?"

This is the question Deutschman poses in Change or Die, and he concludes that although we all have the ability to change our behavior, we rarely ever do. In fact, the odds are 9-to-1 that, when faced with the dire need to change, we won't.

From patients suffering from heart disease to repeat offenders in the criminal justice system to companies trapped in the mold of unsuccessful business practices, to Caregviers destined for failure while reading from the S.C.R.I.P.T. of the "Caregiver's Dilemma," many of us could prevent ominous outcomes by simply changing our mindset. Yet we don't make the change!

Unless that is, we are empowered by three critical key steps; to relate, repeat and reframe our perceptions of the world we live in and how we fit into it.

Change or Die is not about merely reorganizing or restructuring priorities; it's about challenging, inspiring and helping all of us to make the dramatic transformations necessary in any aspect of life— changes that are positive, attainable and absolutely vital.

So how do we do it? Well, to put it simply, we beg borrow and steal from programs like Alcoholics Anonymous and Weight Watchers, but no, we are not changing our name to the Caregiver's Coalition! We are and will remain "Defenders of Caregivers!"

Alcoholics Anonymous and Weight Watchers are so successful because they have adopted these three key elements to change.

Relate: This is about connecting with a person, group, or idea that inspires, motivates and creates in us the possibility, the hope that change is possible.

Repeat: The new behavior needs to be repeated again and again, one day at a time, until it becomes part of us. These new behaviors need to start small so there is a sense of accomplishment that will continue to create hope and motivation.

Reframe: We need to begin to separate from our prior perceptions and reframe our vision of the world and how we are in it.

To be a successful, "Defender of Caregivers," the Caregiver in us must reach out to others and create V.A.L.U.E. Circles where we:

Validate their feelings (but not necessarily their objectivity) of Other Caregivers...

Affirm them as individuals (but not necessarily their conclusions)...

Laugh Lovingly with them (and even AT them, so long as it is Loving)...

Understand and Guide, them (with a pull not a push) to new ways of thinking and seeing...

Empathically and Emphatically (but not blindly) support them!

The Fourth Key Element

For these V.A.L.U.E. Circles to truly work the Caregivers Coalition (nee, the "Defender of Caregivers!") must add a fourth Key element into the equation. The first thing you need to know about this Fourth Key is that it is not fourth; it is FIRST. By addition; when you put it along with Alan Deutschman's pre-existing "Three Keys" it represents "Four Keys" but it is the FIRST Key element and that element is to:

> *Refrain:* from talking about how to be a better Caregiver. When most Caregivers get together, they trade secrets and tips on how to be better Caregivers; they talk about the problems they are having with the people they are Caring for and concentrate on HOW to become a better Caregiver, whereas I want them to focus on WHY they already are Caregivers... instead of focusing on WHO they Care for or HOW they Care for them, we want to explore WHY they Care!

The point behind our V.A.L.U.E. Circle is to immerse ourselves in groups of similar-minded and motivated people where we constantl and consistently remind one another in small yet meaningful ways who, what and why we are Caregivers and that we want (not MUST, but WANT) to view our world in a more positive SELF LOVING way! The focus is on how to be a better individual that is also a Caregiver and not on how to be a better Caregiver.

So, REFRAIN, Relate, Repeat, and Reframe are the Four Keys to form V.A.L.U.E. based relationships that are win-win experiences where it is always BETTER to GIVE and to RECEIVE!

The "Defender of Caregivers!" L.A.W.

Everyone (yes, even you) can become certified as a DOC, a "Defender Of Caregivers" simply by learning, sharing and enforcin the "Defender Of Caregivers" L.A.W. to'

> L – Listen intently

> A – Advise sincerely

> W- Work tirelessly

... to increase Awareness and Acceptance of the Caregiver's Dilemma!

A true "Defender of Caregivers!" will ALWAYS obey the L.A.W.

A true "Defender of Caregivers!" will:

L - Listen intently, to fellow Caregivers who need to vent, share their stories or inquire about their own Caregiver experiences to gain perspective. As an intent listener, a DOC will not interrupt or offer his or her observations until the Caregiver has finished expressing themselves until it is time to...

A - Advise sincerely, based on an unbiased and objective perspective of the Caregiver's plight. The DOC will risk reframing a fellow Caregiver's thinking and perspective if they honestly and objectively consider it to be flawed or DISTORTED and will...

W- Work tirelessly, within an established V.A.L.U.E. Circle to assist their fellow Caregiver to stay true to the mandate of increased AWARENESS and ACCEPTANCE of a fellow Caregiver.

"Defender of Caregivers!" as a PPO

Those of us in Healthcare, and Caregivers in or out of traditional Healthcare, know immediately what a PPO is – it is a Preferred Provider Organization.

In a Preferred Provider Organization, MEMBERS receive discounted medical services so long as they obtain those services and treatment WITHIN the organization. (See Appendix F: PPO)

Well, "Defender of Caregivers!" is a PPO, but it means something different and we are always looking for new MEMBERS! In the world of a "Defender of Caregivers!" MEMBER the initials PPO stand for: Provide, Promote and Obey.

A DOC MEMBER will always seek to help another Caregiver as they:

Provide H.O.P.E

Promote V.A.L.U.E., and

Obey the L.A.W.

CHAPTER 7

How DOC Learned to Accept, Retreat and Surrender... Will YOU?

As we learned in Chapter One of this book, the Caregiver, no matter how tired, stressed or lost they may feel may actually NOT want their duties to end. An end of these duties may signal a partial loss of identity, a loss of a role and of the self-satisfaction derived through the act of Caregiving.

So after hearing this again it will likely not surprise you that I really don't want to see this book come to an end; but Care giving AND writing are temporary. They must end!

Before I leave you I want to reiterate what we accomplished in this book and why it was written and why I think you chose to buy and read it...

YOU MIGHT BE A CAREGIVER *if...*
YOU HAVE LEARNED THE ABILITY TO ACCEPT
YOURSELF THRU AN INCREASED
AWARENESS OF WHO, WHY AND WHAT YOU ARE!

You are a Caregiver whether by Nature (BORN) or Nurture (BORNE) and the hope is that you will use this increased Awareness to Accept yourself as the amazing and perfectly flawed person that you are.

YOU MIGHT BE A NATURAL (BORN) CAREGIVER
(says "Popeye") *if...*
YOU DON'T NEED SOMEONE TO TELL YOU HOW
TO TAKE CARE OF YOURSELF
YOU NEED SOMEONE TO GIVE YOU PERMISSION

I hope in reading this book you know that DOC is here to give you that permission!

YOU MIGHT BE A NURTURE (BORNE) CAREGIVER
(says "Aristotle") *if...*
YOU EMBRACE YOUR EMOTIONS ERGO YOU CAN
HONOR YOURSELF
(AND YOUR EFFORTS) AS YOU CARE FOR OTHERS!

This book is to HONOR you for the commitment you have made, against your Nature, to Nurture and Care for Others.

Further, this book was intended to be a journey of Awareness that will lead whether voluntarily or reluctantly into Acceptance.

There are many amazingly wonderful personality traits associated with being a Caregiver. However, there are also many Cognitive and Emotional traps; if you are not Aware of these inevitabilities; if you do not Accept them as natural, predictable and "normal" you are left alone to analyze and criticize yourself harshly.

Without Awareness and Acceptance you will be perpetually inviting yourself through your own "shouldy attitude" into a party of self-deprecating thoughts instead of learning to relax and enjoy who, what and why you are... and you might continue to "give yourself to *Others* and wonder what happened to YOU!"

So, here it is…

The End…

As I prepared to write the final chapter of this book I sought volunteers to read it and give me some feedback. After speaking with several dozen "volunteers" who endured through the unedited version of this book, I was moved by a letter (and an Essay) I received from Betty R., a self-described "Nature Caregiver!"

In a moment I will share an excerpt of the letter she sent to me after reading this manuscript; but first, allow me to share her personal "thoughts" expressed as a self-portrait in the form of an Essay written several years prior to the creation of "DOC" the "Defender Of Caregivers!"

Why Me?

"It seems that I have been caring for people most of my life. Women by gender give birth and are thought to be naturally the nurturing ones. Yet, many can negate to assume this role of a Caregiver. Is the Caregiver fulfilling their need to be loved, feel important, be in control or are they just extra sensitive to human frailty and want to make things better?

For many years, I wondered my real purpose while here on earth. I thought of myself as "the post" that kept things connected. If I'm the post, then why during a Bernie Siegel lecture… would a self drawing show me to have big shoulders but as the drawing proceeded down the page there was no room left on the page for my feet? His analogy explained that I was not grounded.

So back to the original thoughts, why and who are "the Caregivers?" Perhaps we're just the chosen ones, a difficult task, demanding, leaving one tired and depleted of energy, hoping to make it through by putting one foot in front of the other, thus moving forward."

~ *Betty Ratajczak*

A *"Nature Caregiver" and honorary DOC, "Defender of Caregivers!"*

This is a very profound sharing of "thoughts" by a chronic Natural Caregiver. I know quite a bit about Betty; including her role as a mother and a daughter who has been the primary Caregiver of her own mother for several years.

Her "self portrait" is so typical of the Caregivers I hope to reach here. She sees herself as "the post" that holds Others together; she views herself as having broad shoulders (capable and strong) yet, as Dr. Bernie Siegel advised her, she is not grounded. She is suffering from "the Caregivers Dilemma!"

In addition to her sharing of "thoughts" I also would like to thank Betty for introducing me to the work of Dr. Siegel and his three words of advice on how to approach an illness: accept, retreat and surrender.

Keep in mind that Dr. Siegel is speaking about holistic self-treatment of illness and disease, not Caregiving. And I am not trying to equate being a Caregiver to having an illness or a disease. But I will tell you, they share some of the same symptoms; chronic fatigue, loss of appetite, physical and mental pain, etc...

The following are the words of Dr. Siegel... I took the liberty of changing words such as "illness, disease," etc... and replaced them with phrases like, "being a Caregiver" or "role of a Caregiver." My changes are noted by the [brackets] surrounding them.

I think you will be amazed by how seamlessly it reads with these simple changes.

> You need to accept your situation if you want to be empowered to change it... you need to accept that [being a Caregiver] exists in your life and you are a participant. Once you accept that the [role of Caregiver] has become a part of your life, you can marshal your forces and alter [how it affects you]. If you avoid thinking about it, deny it or feel hopeless, you cannot play a part in changing it and your life.

> Accepting the situation does not mean accepting someone else's prediction about what will happen... No one knows what your future will be... The best course, though, is accepting that you have [burdens, responsibilities, difficulties] while denying anyone's predictions about how your situation will turn out. Individuals are not statistics.

> When I say "retreat," I don't mean withdrawing in the face of a more

powerful opponent. For me a retreat means withdrawing to a quiet place where I can be <u>aware</u> of my thoughts and feelings. The quiet place may be anywhere; the source of true peace and quiet is inside me...

When you have <u>accepted,</u> retreated and prepared yourself to fight, then you are ready to surrender. Again, you do not surrender to outcomes but to events. We waste so much energy fighting the nature of life [and Caregiving]. <u>Accept</u> the nature of life and surrender to it. When you do, you will have peace. When our energy is restored, we stop fighting things we cannot control, and we can start building our lives. Surrender is not about doing nothing; it is about doing the right things.

When you surrender to the [burdens and role of a Caregiver], you continue to [Care for Others], explore your feelings, repair your relationships and do all the other work of healing. But while you are working, you are saying, "Thy will be done" and not "My will be done." Surrender the pain, fear and worries and you'll be able to keep love, hope and joy in your life. As the Serenity Prayer tells us, leave it to God and rest.

Excerpted from Prescriptions for Living
©1998 by Bernie S. Siegel, M.D.,
HarperCollins Publishers, New York, NY

I am quite thankful to both Betty and to Dr. Siegel for this advice to accept, retreat and surrender.

I am comforted in knowing (after already having written this book) that someone so well respected as Dr. Siegel has embraced Acceptance as I have in this book; however, the first challenge is that of Awareness.

No... being a Caregiver is not an illness... but as the saying goes... "the first step is recognizing that you have a problem!"

If you want to learn how to feel better about yourself; how to give to Others without losing yourself; you must first be Aware that you have the tendency to do just that!

You must be aware that you are a pillar (post) without any feet!

I hope throughout this book you have seen, heard and can recognize some things, traits, and tendencies that mirror your own behavior and beliefs.

Throughout this book we offered several "You might be a Caregiver if…" statements… if they gave you a chuckle or an "a-ha Moment" please take it as an invitation to be Aware of the Caregiver in you.

Please learn to EMBRACE these moments by telling yourself, "ah… my Caregiver is showing!" Chuckle at yourself (feel those endorphins) in this moment of Awareness and as Dr. Siegel, and DOC, would suggest, Accept yourself as a perfectly flawed human being.

It is in these moments of Awareness, just like HUMOR (a Healthy Understanding of Matters Others Recognize) that we can more naturally see ourselves as Others see us.

We are not the best judges of ourselves; we must learn to rely on, believe in and Accept the AWE that Others experience when they look at us and our accomplishments. Most of all we must learn that we don't have to Personalize things (Caregiver Distortion #10) and it is ok to say and think…. "I am not sorry you're unhappy!"

In this way we can first HONOR ourselves as we Care for Others!

In closing, let's return to the letter I received from Betty R. after reading the first draft of this book…

Lon, DOC-

I recently read your book… it is good and very insightful.

However, as I was reading it I was thinking, "Yes, this I know. Yet as a Caregiver, how can this help me? We are usually so caught up in the moment there is no time for searching or reading "self-help" books.

My father died 41 years ago. It was a terrible shock and I grieved "poorly." I remember the day of the funeral sitting on the sofa with Mom in our living room. People were leaving the house after saying their goodbyes. I still hear the sound of laughter and seeing an Aunt and two Cousins going down the front steps, leaving to go onto their carefree world. The thought came to me, "today is my day… tomorrow will be theirs." That's the way it is…

In "those days" there wasn't talk of support groups. I'm not sure if I would have attended one???

I suppose that what I'm telling you, at the time of strife, one is

*   *   *

Please join us to share in V.A.L.U.E. – based relationships and discussions on Facebook at "Defender of Caregivers!" Fan Page.

For more information on Lon Kieffer visit him at:
www.LonKieffer.com

For more information on DOC the "Defender of Caregivers!"
visit us at: www.DefenderOfCaregivers.com

Or contact us at: DOC@DefendeOfCaregivers.com

*   *   *

ADDITIONAL READING

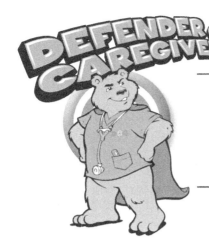

The Story of DOC...

In time you will notice that the "Defending the Caregiver!" philosophy and series of books has two different logos associated with it. The Protected Heart logo and DOC, the "Defender of Caregivers" Bear logo.

There is no great mystery behind this, it just sort of evolved naturally and serendipitously.

DOC the Bear was an amazing coincidence and became a true source of inspiration for Lon Kieffer, the originator of the "Defending the Caregiver!" philosophy.

Lon realized he needed branding and he needed a voice and further, he realized that voice could not and should not always be his own. In time he developed the concept of an "always objective" alter-ego that would see through all of the distorted thinking that Caregivers utilize because they live in a sort of chronic stress by virtue of their empathic way of viewing the world.

But we are getting ahead of ourselves already. Lon approached Greg Cravens, an amazingly talented Cartoonist (trust me, you have seen his work) and asked him , "Draw me a Bear that is a cross between Yogi the Bear and Winnie the Pooh but with Underdog's dundering can-do attitude'"

Ignore for a moment that "dundering" is not actually a word and look at what Greg Cravens drew: The amazing thing about this drawing is that, to this day, Lon and Greg have never met; and at the time they had no idea

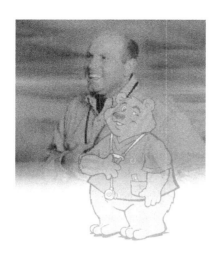

what the other looked like and Greg had never seen this picture.

Above is the picture Lon was using in print media to promote his EnterTraining!"speaking business. At the point of retaining Greg to do these drawings, Lon was seriously considering stopping the "Defender f Caregivers!" project due to costs, schedule and family conflicts. Upon seeing Greg's original drawing of DOC, Lon immediately knew he needed to push forward.

So why a Bear, you ask?

Have you ever seen a mother Bear protect one of her cubs?

You know the reputation. A Bear can be a protective cuddly animal like a big ol' teddy bear or a fierce fighting-mad momma grizzly bear! (Besides, he thought one day DOC might make for a nice little stuffed momento that all his Caregivers would buy as gifts for each other! Not really, but just sayin'.)

DOC can do and say things to and for his Caregivers that a real live human cannot do or say!

Most importantly, DOC is not human!

This is very important! If DOC were human, his Caregivers would be likely to try and take care of him!

Since DOC is a Bear, he can take care of his Caregivers!

DOC can give his Caregivers advice; DOC can fight for them; laugh with them (even laugh at them); cry for them and just be himself with and FOR THEM, his Caregivers!

DOC's most important role in life is to help his Caregivers see and avoid the over utilization of "Cognitive Distortions" as identified by David Burns MD. DOC can help by encouraging you to see things as they are by asking (yes, you guessed it); "What's up DOC?"

He can offer DOC's Orders on a STAT, Daily or PRN basis and frequency. All of DOC's Orders have a duration of: Until Effective. His sincere hope is that his orders will become habit forming!

There are several versions of DOC (and others evolving all the time).

You have already met "Super DOC!" who is supremely confident and always willing to help his Caregivers. He was originally described as; "a cross between Winnie the Pooh and Yogi the Bear but with Underdog's Attitude" (yes, a DOG, not a DOC) that makes him believe he can help everybody even though, in reality, he can't because people have to help themselves. But he sure will try to show the path forward!

Later DOC went through a few modifications where he was tweaked a bit to re-design the Protected Heart Logo (more on that in a moment) as the "O" and DOC was "hard-lined" for re-production purposes.

There is Typical DOC, and Angry DOC in full-blown "Defender" mode. And alas, there is also, Depleted DOC, who is rarely seen publicly but lurks beneath the surface hiding behind a smile and a tough guy exterior only showing himself when he has not benefitted from his own self-defense(s) or when he has failed to accept or recognize that there are other's that are willing to DEFEND him.

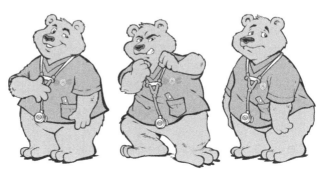

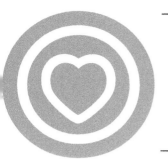

The Protected Heart Logo

Some time ago, Lon Kieffer was honored with a statewide award from the Delaware Health Care Facilities Association when he was recognized as the Administrator of the Year for his work as a Nursing Home Administrator.

His accomplishments at the time were, in his mind, "nothing special," even rather mundane "just doing my job"(DISQUALIFYING THE POSITIVE, Caregiver Distortion #4) because they all had to do with things he did Naturally or felt that the award was a reflection of what his other Caregivers had achieved, such as:

- Industry-leading retention and turnover performance.
- Exceeding financial and regulatory expectations.
- Above industry standard customer and employee satisfaction.
- Industry leading trends in pressure ulcer prevention.

No matter the accomplishment, he discounted it and gave credit to his Caregivers; the women who taught him his original "Get Out of Bed and Go to Work!" philosophy that launched his "EnterTraining!" speaking career.

While at the awards banquet (a banquet where Lon would one day be the keynote speaker and present his program "The Blessings of Long Term Care!" and introduce DOC, the "Defender of Caregivers!" to the world... see a clip here: http://www.youtube.com/user/LonKieffer) Lon sat in the audience and heard over and over again people refer to his profession as a "Heart" business.

He heard Caregiver after Caregiver make reference to how they would "wear my heart on my sleeve" and speak about how vulnerable their feelings were to the circumstances of those they cared for and cared with as he listened he realized that each of these Caregivers had no true insight to the fact that individually and collectively their view on life was that, "They are what they do!"

They had become their profession; their singular and collective outcomes is how they defined their worth and value.

This is known as PERSONALIZATION (Caregiver Distortion #10), where they held themselves responsible for any negative outcomes no matter how ridiculous the notion that they could somehow, through Caregiving, offset the ravages of time and disease or the will of Mother Nature.

He realized that when you put their tendency to "disqualify the positive" (take no credit for good things) on top of "personalization" (accept blame for things beyond their control), you have a toxic "no win" situation where the Caregiver has made an emotionally laden mountain out of the proverbial mole hill AND THIS WAS AT AN AWARDS BANQUET!

Sitting there that night, he found himself with a full blown vision in his head of a heart with protective bands around it... a heart that could give without being harmed. He kept telling himself over and over that until they become AWARE of what they are doing to themselves and ACCEPT that they are doing it... they will continue to be hurt by their efforts.

The more they give, the more they hurt... and the only answer in his mind was AWARENESS and ACCEPTANCE... thus the Protected Heart Logo... heart with two bands of protection.

He also can't help but notice that the Protected Heart Logo also resemble a bull's-eye (and his Caregivers see this first and foremost, as they joke about how often they are targeted by the very people they care for!).

Caregivers are often targeted for the simple nursery school challenge to determine... "which of these things is not like the others, which of these things just doesn't belong?"

Often, Caregivers are the only non-family members present when something very bad or very unexpected happens to a loved one... yes, they get thanks and praise (which they discount immediately... "just doin my job!") but they also get blame and accusations (which they absorb like a sponge... "it was my fault!") as well.

So, where some Caregivers may see a bull's-eye, a target... DOC is offering a Protected Heart and his goal is to make Caregivers AWARE of it and he HOPES they ACCEPT it and learn to HONOR themselves as they Care for Others!

Some of DOC's favorite Quotes & Comments:

The hardest battle you are ever going to fight is the battle to be just you."

~ Leo Buscaglia

DOC-Comment: HONOR <u>yourself</u> as you care for others!

I have found the paradox that if I love until it hurts, then there is no hurt, but only more love.

~ Mother Teresa

Act as if what you do makes a difference. It does.

~ William James

The purpose of life is not to be happy - but to matter, to be productive, to be useful, to have it make some difference that you have lived at all.

~ Leo Rosten

Live simply that others might simply live.

~ Elizabeth Ann Seton

DOC-Comment: Okay, so your ONLY purpose in life... the ONLY reason you are here is so that other's can live! I think Ms. Seton probably enjoyed roller coasters!

We can do no great things, only small things with great love.

~ Mother Teresa

Unless someone like you cares a whole awful lot, nothing is going to get better. It's not.

~ Dr. Seuss

DOC-Comment: Even Dr. Seuss seems to be working against you, perhaps he is not but he seems too. He do! – With apology...DOC!

He who gives when he is asked has waited too long.

~ Sunshine Magazine

DOC-Comment: This sounds directed at the Nurture Caregiver who was BORNE ratherthan BORN into Caregiving...Thank you for being what you were NOT! Thank you for becoming a Caregiver by adopting a new (and more painful) way of thinking and being...Thank you for Caring!

This is the true joy in life - being used for a purpose recognized by

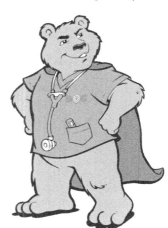

yourself as a mighty one; being thoroughly worn out before you are thrown on the scrap heap; being a force of nature instead of a feverish selfish little clod of ailments and grievances complaining that the world will not devote itself to making you happy.

~ *George Bernard Shaw*

No man stands so straight as when he stoops to help a boy.

~ *Knights of Pythagoras* (Thanks, Jim)

In about the same degree as you are helpful, you will be happy.

~ *Karl Reiland*

We make a living by what we get, but we make a life by what we give.

~ *Winston Churchill*

Service to others is the rent you pay for your room here on earth.

~ *Mohammed Ali*

The first question which the priest and the Levite asked was: "If I stop to help this man, what will happen to me?" But... the good Samaritan reversed the question: "If I do not stop to help this man, what will happen to him?"

~ *Martin Luther King, Jr.*

Here a Nurture Caregiver (Priest and Levite; whose vocation is Caregiving) views helping as a burden or responsibility meets a Nature Caregiver (Good Samaritan; who is

Caregiving naturally) who views it as a Natural obligation where empathy for another is the driving force. Notice; there is no preference here as both Nature and Nurture will help this man!

Nature Caregiver:

Everyone thinks of changing the world, but no one thinks of changing himself.

~ *Leo Nikolaevich Tolstoy*

This is perhaps an insight into the Caregiver's Dilemma. We think we are doing only for and to Others when what we do also affects ourselves! What we do; who we do it for; how often we do it and more importantly WHY we do it has a huge impact on our own feelings of self worth, our own V.A.L.U.E.

Past the seeker as he prayed came the crippled and the beggar and the beaten. And seeing them... he cried, "Great God, how is it that a loving creator can see such things and yet do

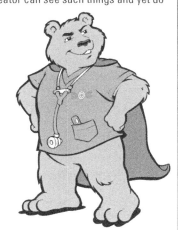

nothing about them?" God said, "I did do something. I made you."

~ Author Unknown

Sometime in your life, hope that you might see one starved man, the look on his face when the bread finally arrives. Hope that you might have baked it or bought or even kneaded it yourself. For that look on his face, for your meeting his eyes across a piece of bread, you might be willing to lose a lot, or suffer a lot, or die a little, even.

~ Daniel Berrigan

Wow! You should "lose a lot, or suffer a lot, or die a little" for others! Now that is a great message for a Caregiver who already is prone to giving too much!

Nurture Caregiver:

The Lord loveth a cheerful giver. He also accepteth from a grouch.

~ Catherine Hall

There is no great sin in recognizing the sacrifices of Caregiving. DOC believes this is actually very healthy! He who gives when he is asked has waited too long.

~Sunshine Magazine

He who gives when he is asked is a Nurture Caregiver; they are BORNE into the Caregiver role by having accepted a burden or responsibility... the Nurture Caregiver should not be judged for having "waited too long" they should be celebrated for having answered the call! This is a classic condemnation that plays on the

vulnerability of Nurture Caregivers! "You should love what you do because you do what you do out of love!" There is nothing wrong with acknowledging, DEFENDing, even Celebrating that you do what you do out of responsibility and in some ways that makes you even more noble than those who have no choice and do so Naturally!

Our prayers for others flow more easily than those for ourselves. This shows we are made to live by charity.

~ C.S.Lewis

What we have done for ourselves alone dies with us; what we have done for others and the world remains and is immortal.

~ Albert Pike (Thanks, Carl)

It's easy to make a buck. It's a lot tougher to make a difference.

~ Tom Brokaw

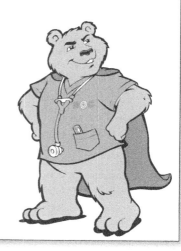

The real question challenge and recommendation for a Caregiver is that it is okay to use a buck to make a difference. The Nature Caregiver doesn't see this; the Nurture Caregiver might! If a service can be paid for with a buck rather than your back... sit down and open your wallet! One must be poor to know the luxury of giving!

~ George Eliot

George...Did you NOT hear what DOC just said? The truth is that "one that is poor must find luxury in giving!" If you can afford God has not called us to see through each other, but to see each other through.

~ Author Unknown

If you have no will to change it, you have no right to criticize it.

~ Author Unknown

This is a bit off topic but I think it is invaluable. If the Caregiver is not willing to change their plight, correct their Dilemma, they ought at lease not criticize themselves for the Dilemma they are in for it is Natural for them; perhaps unavoidable so the self condemnation as a cherry on top is one final slight against themselves. Be ashamed to die until you have won some victory for humanity.

~ Horace Mann

When you dig another out of their troubles, you find a place to bury your own.

~ Author Unknown

It is clearly an inviting and accelerating ride down a steep hill to hide from your own problems (health, financial, relationships) by burying yourself in those of Others! The only gift is a portion of thyself.

~ Ralph Waldo Emerson

Thousands of candles can be lighted from a single candle, and the life of the candle will not be shortened. Happiness never decreases by being shared.

~ Buddha

Not for the Caregiver who seeks their own satisfaction through pleasing Others when they do not establish a fair exchange rate for the V.A.L.U.E. of what they Give and that which they receive. The Caregiver who does not recognize the V.A.L.U.E. of themselves will always be headed for emotional bankruptcy!

Things of the spirit differ from

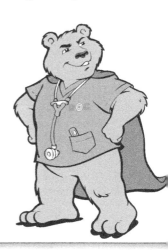

things material in that the more you give the more you have.

~ *Christopher Morley*

It's not that successful people are givers; it is that givers are successful people.

~ *Patti Thor*

Find a need and fill it.

~ *Ruth Stafford Peale*

In giving you are throwing a bridge across the chasm of your solitude.

~ *Antoine de Saint-Exupéry, The Wisdom of the Sands, translated from French by Stuart Gilbert*

Sometimes a man imagines that he will lose himself if he gives himself, and keep himself if he hides himself. But the contrary takes place with terrible exactitude.

~ *Ernest Hello*

You give but little when you give of your possessions. It is when you give of yourself that you truly give.

~ *Kahlil Gibran*

Love never reasons but profusely gives; gives, like a thoughtless prodigal, its all, and trembles lest it has done too little.

~ *Hannah More*

If you have much, give of your wealth; if you have little, give of your heart.

~Arabian Proverb

Bread for myself is a material question. Bread for my neighbor is a spiritual one.

~ *Nicholas Berdyaev*

A bone to the dog is not charity. Charity is the bone shared with the dog, when you are just as hungry as the dog.

~ *Jack London*

If I thought I was going to die tomorrow, I should nevertheless plant a tree today.

~ *Stephan Girard*

I've seen and met angels wearing the disguise of ordinary people living ordinary lives.

~ *Tracy Chapman*

The vicious count their years; virtuous, their acts.

~ *Samuel Johnson*

Look around the habitable world:

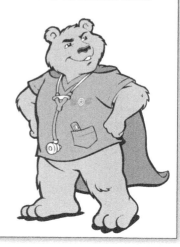

how few Know their own good,
or knowing it, pursue.

~ Juvenal, Satires

The deed is everything,
the glory naught.

~ Johann Wolfgang von Goethe

The great use of life is to spend it for
something that outlasts it.

~ William James

Generosity is not giving me that which
I need more than you do, but it is giving
me that which you
need more than I do.

~ Kahlil Gibran

DOComment: I must be honest! Kahlil
Gibran confuses me but there is some
wisdom in this circular quote. 'Nuff
said? Sometimes, you just gotta
accept that "good enough is good
enough" and let things alone... I will
let this quote alone!

Usefulness is happiness, and... all
other things are but incidental.

~ Lydia Maria Child, The American
Frugal Housewife, 1829

DOComment: This is classic Caregiver
thinking where they confuse their
own V.A.L.U.E. with the usefulness or
service they provide Others; they do
not see their own intrinsic V.A.L.U.E!

What a person believes is not as important as how a person believes.

~ Timothy Virkkala

Go the extra mile. It's never crowded.

~ Author Unknown

DOComment: The journey of a
Caregiver can be lonely and can take
you to places Others have never been!
The key to the DOC Philosophy is to
always be reminded you are NOT
alone; that Others are with you are
your journey even if they are
not visible.

We cannot change anything until
we accept it. Condemnation does
not liberate, it oppresses.

~ C.G. Jung

DOComment: The hallmark of the
DEFENDER philosophy is ACCEPTANCE
and the first step in ACCEPTANCE is
AWARENESS.

If you pursue good with labor, the
labor passes away but the good
remains; if you pursue evil with

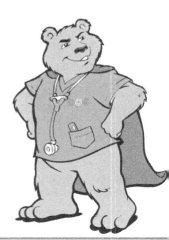

pleasure, the pleasure passes away and the evil remains.

~ *Cicero*

DOComment: For the Caregiver pleasure comes from labor (service to others) and labor, because it is taxing and burdensome is both "good" and "evil" it feels good but it takes a physical and mental toll so… "If you pursue good with labor, the labor passes away but the good remains; if you pursue labor with pleasure, the pleasure passes away and the labor remains."

~ *DOC*
(DOC thinks Cicero would be smiling!)

To put the world right in order, we must first put the nation in order; to put the nation in order, we must first put the family in order; to put the family in order, we must first cultivate our personal life; we must first set our hearts right.

~ *Confucius*

Every man feels instinctively that all the beautiful sentiments in the world weigh less than a single lovely action.

~ *Lowell*

You can't lead anyone else further than you have gone yourself. ~Gene Mauch
If everyone howled at every injustice, every act of barbarism, every act of unkindness, then we would be taking the first step towards a real humanity.

~ *Nelson DeMille*

My piece of bread only belongs to me when I know that everyone else

has a share, and that no one starves while I eat.

~ *Leo Tolstoy*

If you think you are too small to be effective, you have never been in bed with a mosquito.

~ *Betty Reese*

There is no use whatever trying to help people who do not help themselves. You cannot push anyone up a ladder unless he is willing to climb himself.

~ *Andrew Carnegie*

Let no one ever come to you without leaving better and happier.

~ *Mother Teresa*

When I was a young man, I wanted to change the world. I found it was difficult to change the world, so I tried to change my nation. When I found I couldn't change the nation, I began to

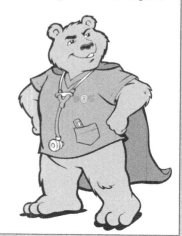

focus on my town. I couldn't
change the town and as an older
man, I tried to change my family.
Now, as an old man, I realize the only
thing I can change is myself, and
suddenly I realize that if long ago I had
changed myself, I could have made
an impact on my family. My family
and I could have made an impact on
our town. Their impact could have
changed the nation and I could indeed
have changed the world.

~ Author Unknown

Everybody can be great. Because
anybody can serve. You don't have to
have a college degree to serve. You
don't have to make your subject and
your verb agree to serve.... You don't
have to know the second theory of
thermodynamics in physics to serve.
You only need a heart full of grace.
A soul generated by love.

~Martin Luther King, Jr.

Find out how much God has given
you and from it take what you need;
the remainder is needed by others.

~ Saint Augustine

* * *

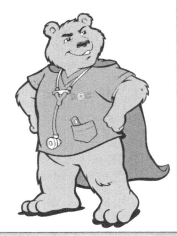

APPENDIX

Appendix A: Myers-Briggs

Since its inception in 1963 the Myers-Briggs Type Indicator (MBTI) has been the industry standard used to determine "Personality Type" in professional and social settings.

Isabel Briggs Myers, with a bachelor's degree in political science and no academic affiliation yet was responsible for the creation of what has become the most widely used and highly respected personality inventory of all time.

The following excerpt of "The Story of Isabel Briggs-Myers" is taken from the Center for Applications of Psychological Type's official website: http://www.capt.org/mbti-assessment isabel-myers.htm

> The Myers-Briggs Type Indicator® (MBTI®) instrument, now taken by at least two million people each year-and translated into sixteen languages-was developed over a period of more than forty years, progressing from Isabel Myers' dining room to a cottage industry, to the prestigious Educational Testing Service, and to its current publisher, CPP, Inc.
>
> Isabel Myers and her mother, Katharine Cook Briggs, both astute observers of human behavior, were drawn to C. G. Jung's work, which sparked their interest into a passionate devotion to put the theory of psychological type to practical use.
>
> With the onset of World War II, Isabel Myers recognized that a psychological instrument that has as its foundation the understanding and appreciation of human differences would be invaluable. She researched and developed the Indicator over the next four decades, until her death in 1980. Following are the tenets of Isabel Myers' philosophy, found among her papers after her death. She was known for her keen intelligence and tenacious curiosity, as well as a deeply held set of values and generosity of spirit. She is remembered for her enormous contribution to the field of psychological testing and to the theory of typology, but also for her strength of character and her tireless pursuit of human understanding.

What Is To Be Desired?

Self-respect:	*To be part of the solution, not part of the problem*
Love:	*To love the human beings that mean the most to me, and contribute to their lives if I can*
Peace of Mind:	*To avoid mistakes that make me regret the past or fear the future*
Involvement:	*Always to be tremendously interested*
Understanding:	*To incorporate the things, people and ideas that happen to me into a coherent concept of the world*
Freedom:	*To work at what interests me most, with minimum expenditure of time and energy on non-essentials*

~ Isabel Briggs Myers

Much of the following is excerpted from Wikipedia and is offered in an effort of expediency a more detailed and thorough understanding of the MBTI can be obtained through a simple internet search.

The Myers-Briggs Type Indicator (MBTI) assessment is a psychometric questionnaire designed to measure psychological in how people perceive the world and make decisions. These preferences were extrapolated from the typologi-

cal theories proposed by Carl Gustav Jung and first published in his 1921 book Psychological Types (English edition, 1923).

he original developers of the personality inventory were Katharine Cook Briggs and her aughter, Isabel Briggs Myers. They began creating the indicator during World War II, elieving that a knowledge of personality preferences would help women who were entering 1e industrial workforce for the first time to identify the sort of war-time jobs where they vould be "most comfortable and effective".[1]:xiii The initial questionnaire grew into the 1yers-Briggs Type Indicator, which was first published in 1962. The MBTI focuses on normal opulations and emphasizes the value of naturally occurring differences.[3]

PP Inc., the publisher of the MBTI instrument, calls it "the world's most widely used person-lity assessment",[4] with as many as two million assessments administered annually. The PP and other proponents state that the indicator meets or exceeds the reliability of other sychological instruments[5][6] and cite reports of individual behavior.[7] Some studies have ound strong support for construct validity, internal consistency, and test-retest reliability, al-lough variation was observed.[8][9] However, some academic psychologists have criticized 1e MBTI instrument, claiming that it "lacks convincing validity data".[10][11][12][13] Some tudies have shown the statistical validity and reliability to be low.[13][14][15] The use of the 1yers-Briggs Type Indicator as a predictor of job success has not been supported in stud-es,[15][16] and its use for this purpose is expressly discouraged in *The Manual*.[17]

he definitive published source of reference for the Myers-Briggs Type Indicator is *The Manual* produced by CPP.[18] However, the registered trademark rights to the terms *Myers-riggs Type Indicator and MBTI* have been assigned from the publisher to the Myers-Briggs ype Indicator Trust.

ONCEPTS

s the MBTI *Manual* states, the indicator "is designed to implement a theory; therefore the 1eory must be understood to understand the MBTI"[1]

undamental to the Myers-Briggs Type Indicator is the theory of psychological type as riginally developed by Carl Jung.[1]:xiii Jung proposed the existence of two dichotomous airs of cognitive functions:

he "rational" (judging) functions: *thinking and feeling*

he "irrational" (perceiving) functions: *sensing and intuition*

ung went on to suggest that these functions are expressed in either an introverted or xtraverted form.[1]:17 From Jung's original concepts, Briggs and Myers developed their own 1eory of psychological type, described below, on which the MBTI is based.

YPE

ung's typological model regards psychological type as similar to left or right handedness: 1dividuals are either born with, or develop, certain preferred ways of thinking and acting. he MBTI sorts some of these psychological differences into four opposite pairs, or ichotomies, with a resulting 16 possible psychological types. None of these types are *better* r *worse*; however, Briggs and Myers theorized that individuals naturally *prefer* one overall ombination of type differences. In the same way that writing with the left hand is hard work for a right-hander, so people tend to find using their opposite psychological preferences more difficult, even if they can become more proficient (and therefore behaviorally flexible) with practice and development.

The 16 types are typically referred to by an abbreviation of four letters—the initial letters of each of their four type preferences (except in the case of *intuition*, which uses the abbreviation *N* to distinguish it from Introversion). For instance:

ESTJ: extraversion (E), sensing (S), thinking (T), judgment (J)
INFP: introversion (I), intuition (N), feeling (F), perception (P)

And so on for all 16 possible type combinations.

Four Dichotomies

Dichotomies
Extraversion (**E**) - (**I**) Introversion
Sensing (**S**) - (**N**) Intuition
Thinking (**T**) - (**F**) Feeling
Judgment (**J**) - (**P**) Perception

The four pairs of preferences or *dichotomies* are shown in the table above.

Note that the terms used for each dichotomy have specific technical meanings relating to the MBTI which differ from their everyday usage. For example, people who prefer judgment over perception are not necessarily more *judgmental* or *less perceptive*. Nor does the MBTI instrument measure aptitude; it simply indicates for one preference over another. [17]:3 Someone reporting a high score for extraversion over introversion cannot be correctl described as *more* extraverted: they simply have a clear *preference*.

Point scores on each of the dichotomies can vary considerably from person to person, even among those with the same type. However, Isabel Myers considered the *direction* of the preference (for example, E vs. I) to be more important than the *degree* of the preference (for example, very clear vs. slight). The expression of a person's psychological type is more than the sum of the four individual preferences. The preferences interact through type dynamics and type development.

ATTITUDES: EXTRAVERSION (E)/INTROVERSION (I)

Myers-Briggs literature uses the terms *extraversion* and *introversion* as Jung first used them. Extraversion means "outward-turning" and introversion means "inward-turning." These specific definitions vary somewhat from the popular usage of the words. Note that *extraversion* is the spelling used in MBTI publications.

The preferences for extraversion and introversion are often called as attitudes. Briggs and Myers recognized that each of the cognitive functions can operate in the external world of behavior, action, people, and things (*extraverted attitude*) or the internal world of ideas and reflection (*introverted attitude*). The MBTI assessment sorts for an overall preference for or or the other.

People who prefer extraversion draw energy from action: they tend to act, then reflect, then act further. If they are inactive, their motivation tends to decline. To rebuild their energy, extraverts need breaks from time spent in reflection. Conversely, those who prefer introversion *expend* energy through action: they prefer to reflect, then act, then reflect agai

106

To rebuild their energy, introverts need quiet time alone, away from activity.

The extravert's flow is directed outward toward people and objects, and the introvert's is directed inward toward concepts and ideas. Contrasting characteristics between extraverts and introverts include the following:

- Extraverts are *action* oriented, while introverts are *thought* oriented.

- Extraverts seek *breadth* of knowledge and influence, while introverts seek *depth* of knowledge and influence.

- Extraverts often prefer more *frequent* interaction, while introverts prefer more *substantial* interaction.

- Extraverts recharge and get their energy from spending time with *people*, while introverts recharge and get their energy from spending time *alone*.

FUNCTIONS: SENSING (S)/INTUITION (N) AND THINKING (T)/FEELING (F)

Jung identified two pairs of psychological functions:

- The two *perceiving* functions, sensing and intuition

- The two *judging* functions, thinking and feeling

According to the Myers-Briggs typology model, each person uses one of these four functions more dominantly and proficiently than the other three; however, all four functions are used at different times depending on the circumstances.

Sensing and *intuition* are the information-gathering (perceiving) functions. They describe how new information is understood and interpreted. Individuals who prefer *sensing* are more likely to trust information that is in the present, tangible and concrete: that is, information that can be understood by the five senses. They tend to distrust hunches, which seem to come "out of nowhere."[1]:2 They prefer to look for details and facts. For them, the meaning is in the data. On the other hand, those who prefer *intuition* tend to trust information that is more abstract or theoretical, that can be associated with other information (either remembered or discovered by seeking a wider context or pattern). They may be more interested in future possibilities. They tend to trust those flashes of insight that seem to bubble up from the unconscious mind. The meaning is in how the data relates to the pattern or theory.

Thinking and *feeling* are the decision-making (judging) functions. The thinking and feeling functions are both used to make rational decisions, based on the data received from their information-gathering functions (sensing or intuition). Those who prefer *thinking* tend to decide things from a more detached standpoint, measuring the decision by what seems reasonable, logical, causal, consistent and matching a given set of rules. Those who prefer *feeling* tend to come to decisions by associating or empathizing with the situation, looking at it 'from the inside' and weighing the situation to achieve, on balance, the greatest harmony, consensus and fit, considering the needs of the people involved.

As noted already, people who prefer thinking do not necessarily, in the everyday sense, "think better" than their feeling counterparts; the opposite preference is considered an equally rational way of coming to decisions (and, in any case, the MBTI assessment is a measure of preference, not ability). Similarly, those who prefer feeling do not necessarily have "better" emotional reactions than their thinking counterparts.

DOMINANT FUNCTION

According to Myers and Briggs, people use all four cognitive functions. However, one function is generally used in a more conscious and confident way. This dominant function is supported by the secondary (auxiliary) function, and to a lesser degree the tertiary function. The fourth and least conscious function is always the opposite of the dominant function. Myers called this inferior function the *shadow*.

The four functions operate in conjunction with the attitudes (extraversion and introversion). Each function is used in either an extraverted or introverted way. A person whose dominant function is extraverted intuition, for example, uses intuition very differently from someone whose dominant function is introverted intuition.

LIFESTYLE: JUDGMENT (J)/PERCEPTION (P)

Myers and Briggs added another dimension to Jung's typological model by identifying that people also have a preference for using either the *judging* function (thinking or feeling) or their *perceiving* function (sensing or intuition) when relating to the outside world (extraversion).

Myers and Briggs held that types with a preference for *judgment* show the world their preferred judging function (thinking or feeling). So TJ types tend to appear to the world as logical, and FJ types as empathetic. According to Myers, judging types like to "have matters settled."

Those types who prefer perception show the world their preferred *perceiving* function (sensing or intuition). So SP types tend to appear to the world as concrete and NP types as abstract. According to Myers, perceptive types prefer to "keep decisions open."

For extraverts, the J or P indicates their *dominant* function; for introverts, the J or P indicates their *auxiliary* function. Introverts tend to show their dominant function outwardly only in matters "important to their inner worlds." For example:

Because ENTJ types are extraverts, the J indicates that their *dominant* function is their preferred judging function (extraverted thinking). ENTJ types introvert their auxiliary perceiving function (introverted intuition). The tertiary function is sensing and the inferior function is introverted feeling.

Because INTJ types are introverts, the J indicates that their *auxiliary* function is their preferred judging function (extraverted thinking). INTJ types introvert their dominant perceiving function (introverted intuition). The tertiary function is feeling, and the inferior function is extraverted sensing.

Appendix B: Nature vs. Nurture

The **nature versus nurture** debate concerns the relative importance of an individual's innate qualities ("nature," i.e. nativism, or innatism) versus personal experiences ("nurture," i.e. empiricism or behaviorism) in determining or causing individual differences in physical and behavioral traits.

"Nature versus nurture" in its modern sense was coined[1][2][3] by the English Victorian polymath Francis Galton in discussion of the influence of heredity and environment on social advancement, although the terms had been contrasted previously, for example by Shakespeare (in his play, *The Tempest*: 4.1). Galton was influenced[4] by the book *On the Origin of Species* written by his cousin, Charles Darwin. The concept embodied in the phrase has been criticized[3][4] for its binary simplification of two tightly interwoven parameters, as for example an environment of wealth, education and social privilege are often historically passed to genetic offspring.

The view that humans acquire all or almost all their behavioral traits from "nurture" is known as tabula rasa ("blank slate"). This question was once considered to be an appropriate division of developmental influences, but since both types of factors are known to play such interacting roles in development, many modern psychologists consider the question naive—representing an outdated state of knowledge.

In the social and political sciences, the nature versus nurture debate may be contrasted with the structure versus agency debate (i.e. socialization versus individual autonomy).

SCIENTIFIC APPROACH

To disentangle the effects of genes and environment, behavioral geneticists perform adoption and twin studies. These seek to decompose the variance (differences) in a population into genetic and environmental components. This move from individuals to populations makes a critical difference in the way we think about nature and nurture. This difference is perhaps highlighted in the quote attributed to Psychologist Donald Hebb who is said to have once answered a journalist's question of "which, nature or nurture, contributes more to personality?" by asking in response, "Which contributes more to the area of a rectangle, its length or its width?"]For a particular rectangle, its area is indeed the product of its length and width. Moving to a population, however, this analogy masks the fact that there are many individuals, and that it is meaningful to talk about their differences. Thus if a game such as soccer defined the width of a playing field very tightly, but left the length unspecified, then differences in the area of the playing fields would be almost entirely due to differences in length.

Scientific approaches also seek to break down variance beyond these two categories of nature and nurture. Thus rather than "nurture", behavior geneticists distinguish shared family factors (i.e., those shared by siblings, making them more similar) and nonshared factors (i.e., those that uniquely affect individuals, making siblings different). To express the portion of the variance due to the "nature" component, behavioral geneticists generally refer to the heritability of a trait.

With regard to the Big Five personality traits as well as adult IQ in the general U.S. population, the portion of the overall variance that can be attributed to shared family effects is often negligible.[11] On the other hand, most traits are thought to be at least partially heritable. In this context, the "nature" component of the variance is generally thought to be more important than that ascribed to the influence of family upbringing.

In her Pulitzer Prize-nominated book *The Nurture Assumption*, author Judith Harris argues that "nurture," as traditionally defined in terms of family upbringing does not effectively explain the variance for most traits (such as adult IQ and the Big Five personality traits) in the general population of the United States. On the contrary, Harris suggests that either peer groups or random environmental factors (i.e., those that are independent of family upbringing) are more important than family environmental effects.[12][13]

Although "nurture" has historically been referred to as the care given to children by the parents, with the mother playing a role of particular importance, this term is now regarded by some as any environmental (not genetic) factor in the contemporary *nature versus nurture* debate. Thus the definition of "nurture" has expanded to include influences on development arising from prenatal, parental, extended family, and peer experiences, and extending to influences such as media, marketing, and socio-economic status. Indeed, a substantial source of environmental input to human nature may arise from stochastic variations in prenatal development.[14][15]

Appendix C: Cognitive Distortions

COGNITIVE DISTORTION (compliments of Wikipedia)

Cognitive distortions are exaggerated and irrational thoughts identified in cognitive therapy and its variants, which in theory perpetuate certain psychological disorders. The theory of cognitive distortions was first proposed by David D. Burns, MD. Eliminating these distortions and negative thoughts is said to improve mood and discourage maladies such as depression and chronic anxiety. The process of learning to refute these distortions is called "cognitive restructuring."

LIST OF DISTORTIONS

Many cognitive distortions are also logical fallacies;

1. **All-or-nothing thinking (splitting)** – Thinking of things in absolute terms, like "always", "every", "never", and "there is no alternative". Few aspects of human behavior are so absolute. (See false dilemma.) All-or-nothing-thinking can contribute to depression. (See depression). Also called dichotomous thinking.

2. **Overgeneralization** – Taking isolated cases and using them to make wide generalizations. (See hasty generalization.)

3. **Mental filter** – Focusing almost exclusively on certain, usually negative or upsetting, aspects of an event while ignoring other positive aspects. For example, focusing on a tiny imperfection in a piece of otherwise useful clothing. (See misleading vividness.)

4. **Disqualifying the positive** – Continually deemphasizing or "shooting down" positive experiences for arbitrary, ad hoc reasons. (See special pleading.)

5. **Jumping to conclusions** – Drawing conclusions (usually negative) from little (if any) evidence. Two specific subtypes are also identified:

   - *Mind reading* – Assuming special knowledge of the intentions or thoughts of others.

   - *Fortune telling* – Exaggerating how things will turn out before they happen. (See slippery slope.)

6. **Magnification and minimization** – Distorting aspects of a memory or situation through magnifying or minimizing them such that they no longer correspond to objective reality. This is common enough in the normal population to popularize idioms such as "make a mountain out of a molehill." In depressed clients, often the positive characteristics of other people are exaggerated and negative characteristics are understated. There is one subtype of magnification:

   - *Catastrophizing* – Focusing on the worst possible outcome, however unlikely, or thinking that a situation is unbearable or impossible when it is really just uncomfortable.

7. **Emotional reasoning** – Making decisions and arguments based on intuitions or personal feeling rather than an objective rationale and evidence. (See appeal to consequences.)

8. **Should statements** – Patterns of thought which imply the way things "should" or "ought" to be rather than the actual situation the patient is faced

111

with, or having **rigid rules** which the patient believes will "always apply" no matter what the circumstances are. Albert Ellis termed this "Musturbation". (See wishful thinking.)

9.   **Labeling and mislabeling** – Explaining behaviors or events, merely by naming them; related to overgeneralization. Rather than describing the specific behavior, a patient assigns a label to someone or himself that implies absolute and unalterable terms. Mislabeling involves describing an event with language that is highly colored and emotionally loaded.

10. **Personalization** – Attribution of personal responsibility (or causal role) for events over which the patient has no control. This pattern is also applied to others in the attribution of blame.

NOTE: Dr. Burns is silent on the issue of how his Cognitive Distortions become Caregiver Distortions in the humble and anecdotal opinion of DOC.

Appendix D: Antagonyms (official and unofficial)

Antagonyms are words that can mean the opposite of itself... here are some official and UNOFFICIAL examples:

bad (that was a bad movie)
BAD (that movie was BAD!)

bound (bound for Chicago, moving)
bound (tied up, unable to move)

cleave (to cut apart)
cleave (to seal together)

buckle (buckle your pants -- to hold together)
buckle (knees buckled -- to collapse, fall aprt)

citation (award for good behavior)
citation (penalty for bad behavior)

clip (attach to)
clip (cut off from)

cut (get into a line)
cut (get out of a class)

dust (remove dust)
dust (apply dust -- fingerprints)

fast (moving rapidly)
fast (fixed in position)

give (meaning to give to others)
GIVE (meaning to GET for a Caregiver!)

left (remaining)
left (having gone)

literally (literally)
literally (figuratively)

moot (arguable)
moot (not worthy of argument)

oversight (watchful control)
oversight (something not noticed)

sick (I don't feel good, I am sick)
SICK (that basketball move SICK!)

Appendix E: Aristotle (courtesy of Wikipedia)

Aristotle (Greek: , *Aristotél s*) (384 BC – 322 BC)[1] was a Greek philosopher, a student of Plato and teacher of Alexander the Great. His writings cover many subjects, including physics, metaphysics, poetry, theater, music, logic, rhetoric, linguistics, politics, government, ethics, biology, and zoology. Together with Plato and Socrates (Plato's teacher), Aristotle is one of the most important founding figures in Western philosophy. Aristotle's writings were the first to create a comprehensive system of Western philosophy, encompassing morality and aesthetics, logic and science, politics and metaphysics.

Aristotle's views on the physical sciences profoundly shaped medieval scholarship, and their influence extended well into the Renaissance, although they were ultimately replaced by Newtonian physics. In the zoological sciences, some of his observations were confirmed to be accurate only in the 19th century. His works contain the earliest known formal study of logic, which was incorporated in the late 19th century into modern formal logic. In metaphysics, Aristotelianism had a profound influence on philosophical and theological thinking in the Islamic and Jewish traditions in the Middle Ages, and it continues to influence Christian theology, especially the scholastic tradition of the Catholic Church. His ethics, though always influential, gained renewed interest with the modern advent of virtue ethics. All aspects of Aristotle's philosophy continue to be the object of active academic study today. Though Aristotle wrote many elegant treatises and dialogues (Cicero described his literary style as "a river of gold"), it is thought that the majority of his writings are now lost and only about one-third of the original works have survived.

Appendix F: Preferred Provider Organization

In health insurance in the United States, a **preferred provider organization** (or "PPO", sometimes referred to as a *participating* **provider organization** or **preferred provider option**) is a managed care organization of medical doctors, hospitals, and other health care providers who have covenanted with an insurer or a third-party administrator to provide health care at reduced rates to the insurer's or administrator's clients.

OVERVIEW

A preferred provider organization is a subscription-based medical care arrangement. A membership allows a substantial discount below the regularly charged rates of the designated professionals partnered with the organization. Preferred provider organizations themselves earn money by charging an access fee to the insurance company for the use of their network (unlike the usual insurance with premiums and corresponding payments paid either in full or partially by the insurance provider to the medical doctor). They negotiate with providers to set fee schedules, and handle disputes between insurers and providers. PPOs can also contract with one another to strengthen their position in certain geographic areas without forming new relationships directly with providers. This will be mutually beneficial in theory, as the insurer will be billed at a reduced rate when its insureds utilize the services of the "preferred" provider and the provider will see an increase in its business as almost all and or insureds in the organization will use only providers who are members. PPOs have gained popularity in the past decade because, although they tend to have slightly higher premiums than HMOs and other more restrictive plans, they offer patients more flexibility overall.

PPO

Other features of a preferred provider organization generally include utilization review, where representatives of the insurer or administrator review the records of treatments provided to verify that they are appropriate for the condition being treated rather than largely or solely being performed to increase the amount of reimbursement due. Another near-universal feature is a pre-certification requirement, in which scheduled (non-emergency) hospital admissions and, in some instances outpatient surgery as well, must have prior approval of the insurer and often undergo "utilization review" in advance

Appendix G:

Caregiver Affirmations (compliments of Kid Planet.org)

I forgive myself and others, I live in trust for the future, and I embrace this moment of life.

I take time to cherish myself and to enjoy life, to accept the support and company of others.

I accept the mystery of life and suffering, and I know that the important gift I give is my healing love and caring, listening presence.

I eat well, I exercise, I get enough sleep, and I speak kindly to myself.

I keep a sense of humor and live life in gratefulness for all the small gifts of life, and I am open to my source of power beyond myself.

I set limits with people and make my own needs and feelings known to others.

I am a wonderful source of healing for those that I care for because I first love and care for myself.

DOC's Affirmations:

I am AWARE of who I am and I ACCEPT and embrace myself and the help of Others; I will HONOR myself as I care for Others!

I have and provide H.O.P.E. to and for Others; I seek and promote relationships of V.A.L.U.E.; obey the L.A.W.

Appendix H:

How to become an AWESOME HUMAN BEING (a continual work in progress)

~ A lesson from the "Get Out of Bed and Go to Work" Philosophy

What is it that attracts people to a job in healthcare? The old adage is that, "they want to help people." Not true! The truth is most of us just want a job! The paradox is that to keep their job and to be effective and satisfied in their job, they must help people.

Why do some of us WANT to "Get Out of Bed and Go to Work!" while others simply manage to do so? How is it that some of us can help our patients and our organization by giving of ourselves and feel nurtured in the process while others give of themselves only to feel depleted?

I have been a HealthCare warrior for over 25 years and at various times along the way I have been on both sides of this equation. Once I slowed down long enough to recognize the things in common among those who not only survived, but thrived in this emotionally and physically challenging environment I started to identify some common traits. Along the way I discovered several secrets to success. Through my speaking and consulting I have branded these secrets under the philosophy of "Get Out of Bed and Go To Work!"

I enjoy sharing these AWESOME secrets with you (after all, a secret is best once it has been shared) through my Love, Laugh and Learn Lectures. You've heard of the 80/20 rule (the "Pareto" principle) where 80% of the problem is caused by 20% of the people? You remember biblical lessons by numbered passages. Numbers are powerful!

Here is my 10 – 3 – 2 – 1 Principle of "Get Out of Bed and Go to Work!": Ten stands for unattainable perfection so far away that we should only hold it as a vision; a promised land, and 3-2-1 represents the self-awareness process of counting down to where we start on our journey TOGETHER TODAY!

Here is the form of the 10-3-2-1 Secrets I share in live programs; THE:

- Ten Commandments of "Get Out of Bed and Go to Work!"

- Three Step "How To" Manual of "Get Out of Bed and Go to Work!"

- Two Steps of "How to Get People to Jump Through Hoops"

AND - - -

- ONE Guiding Affirmation: "If you cannot Laugh at (or Care for) yourself; You have no right to Laugh at (or Care for) others!"

Along the way I will invite you to become a member of GOOBERS Nation! How do you join GOOBERS? You simply commit to: Get Out Of Bed, Everyday, Rise and Shine! If ever you need help with this, please call: 1-888-GOOBERZ (hey, the S wasn't available; an example of acceptance: the first principal of becoming AWESOME!).

I will even give you a gentle push in the form of a Helping Human HAND; not just one hand but all FIVE FINGERS! Just like fruits and vegetables all five are ESSENTIAL to healthy living and thriving as a healthcare HUMAN BEING. The ones that thrive have all five!

Five Essential Fingers of a Helping HUMAN Hand

1. ***H**andle Negativity (people and situations)* – There are nasty people, personalities and attitudes everywhere you go in all walks of life; and difficult situations are inevitable. GOOBERS never <u>allow these situations to fester and grow!</u> GOOBERS address negativity immediately using natural yet

effective techniques (a sense of humor; sincerity; to turn these incidents into opportunities. They never avoid them or feed into them just to survive the moment.

2.   *Understand Success* (*and define: CARE*) How do we define success in Healthcare? Dictionary.com defines CARE for others as: *serious attention and protection.* We must all learn that CARE is a model of independence NOT dependence. Our role is one of support, concern and protection, NOT doing things for others that they can do for themselves. Success as an organization depends on satisfying the customer; rewarding and supporting co-workers; and achieving a profit (monetarily or by reputation) for the company. We must Understand and Accept things as they actually are; this is a three legged stool and a failure in any one area leaves us with no place to sit.

3.   *Motivate Yourself Daily* There is no substitute for this; you must "Get Out of Bed and Go to Work!" all by yourself. If you cannot take care of yourself, you have no right to take care of others! We can be happy anywhere and always or nowhere and never. To be a successful HUMAN BEING you have one AwESOME responsibility and Expectation and that is the genuine desire to improve your life and the lives of those you touch. GOOBER Commandment #5: You must be inspired by what you are trying to do!

4.   *Add Value* to your organization as a measure of your own achievements. If you are motivated to help people you must recognize that if you are not helping your organization along the way, you will not continue to have the opportunity to do what you love. If you are motivated simply to bring home a paycheck; the same rule applies. You must add value to the organization.

5.   *Notice and Notify Successes (of Yourself and of Others)!* This is the FIFTH finger of the Human Hand. Any trained animal can demonstrate a certain level of achievement in the previous four (in fact; the training process of rewards and withholding rewards relies upon this) but the ability to notice and reward yourself and those around you is truly a human attribute; it is the proverbial thumb of evolution allowing a team to succeed. Commandment number eight says; "Thou Shalt Take your Successes Where You Find Them!" You must reward yourself and those around you. There is no "higher authority" or "chain of command" when it comes to acknowledgement and praise. Applause is spontaneous and comes from any-and-all in attendance but it takes at least two hands to make the noise.

So, whether you use your HUMAN hand to help (and CARE for) others or to hold it out to accept a paycheck really does not matter. We need you on the team either way. But for nurturing rather than compensation what truly matters is that you accept the AWESOME responsibility and privilege to touch others and affect their lives using your HUMAN HAND because you are a HUMAN BEING, BEING HUMAN. That is what GOOBERS do and it is AWESOME!

Thank you for what you do and for allowing me to do what I do!

Please do not hesitate to call me if I can be of any assistance to you as you

Love, Laugh and Learn along Life's Journey!

Lon@LonKieffer.com • 1 (888) GOOBERZ • 1 (888) 466-2379 • www.LonKieffer.com

Appendix I: Empathy (compliments of Wikipedia)

Empathy

Empathy is the capacity to recognize and, to some extent, share feelings (such as sadness or happiness) that are being experienced by another sentient or semi-sentient being. Someone may need to have a certain amount of empathy before they are able to feel compassion.

Theorists and definition

Empathy is an ability with many different definitions. They cover a broad spectrum, ranging from feeling a concern for other people that creates a desire to help them, experiencing emotions that match another person's emotions, knowing what the other person is thinking or feeling, to blurring the line between self and other.[5] Below is a list of various definitions of empathy:

- Daniel Batson: "A motivation oriented towards the other."[6]

- D. M. Berger: "The capacity to know emotionally what another is experiencing from within the frame of reference of that other person, the capacity to sample the feelings of another or to put one's self in another's shoes."[7]

- Jean Decety: *A sense of similarity in feelings experienced by the self and the other, without confusion between the two individuals.Decety, J., & Jackson, P.L. (2004). The functional architecture of human empathy. Behavioral and Cognitive Neuroscience Reviews, 3, 71-100[8]*

- Nancy Eisenberg: *An affective response that stems from the apprehension or comprehension of another's emotional state or condition, and that is similar to what the other person is feeling or would be expected to feel.[9]*

- R. R. Greenson: To empathize means to share, to experience the feelings of another person.[citation needed]

- Alvin Goldman: "The ability to put oneself into the mental shoes of another person to understand her emotions and feelings."[10]

- Martin Hoffman: any process where the attended perception of the object's state generates a state in the subject that is more applicable to the object's state or situation than to the subject's own prior state or situation. [citation needed]

- William Ickes: A complex form of psychological inference in which observation, memory, knowledge, and reasoning are combined to yield insights into the thoughts and feelings of others.[citation needed]

- Heinz Kohut: Empathy is the capacity to think and feel oneself into the inner life of another person[11]

- Carl Rogers: To perceive the internal frame of reference of another with accuracy and with the emotional components and meanings which pertain thereto as if one were the person, but without ever losing the "as if" condition. Thus, it means to sense the hurt or the pleasure of another as he senses it and to perceive the causes thereof as he perceives them, but without ever losing the recognition that it is as if I were hurt or pleased and so forth.[12]

- Roy Schafer: Empathy involves the inner experience of sharing in and comprehending the momentary psychological state of another person.[13]

- Wynn Schwartz: We recognize others as empathic when we feel that they have accurately acted on or somehow acknowledged in stated or unstated fashion our values or motivations, our knowledge, and our skills or competence, but especially as they appear to recognize the significance of our actions in a manner that we can tolerate their being recognized.[14]

- Edith Stein: Empathy is the experience of foreign consciousness in general.[15]

- Simon Baron-Cohen (2003): Empathy is about spontaneously and naturally tuning into the other person's thoughts and feelings, whatever these might be [...]There are two major elements to empathy. The first is the cognitive component: Understanding the others feelings and the ability to take their perspective [...] the second element to empathy is the affective component. This is an observer's appropriate emotional response to another person's emotional state.[16]

- Khen Lampert (2005): "[Empathy] is what happens to us when we leave our own bodies...and find ourselves either momentarily or for a longer period of time in the mind of the other. We observe reality through her eyes, feel her emotions, share in her pain."[17]

Since empathy involves understanding the emotional states of other people, the way it is characterized is derivative of the way emotions themselves are characterized. If, for example, emotions are taken to be centrally characterized by bodily feelings, then grasping the bodily feelings of another will be central to empathy. On the other hand, if emotions are more centrally characterized by a combination of beliefs and desires, then grasping these beliefs and desires will be more essential to empathy. The ability to imagine oneself as another person is a sophisticated imaginative process. However the basic capacity to recognize emotions is probably innate[citation needed] and may be achieved unconsciously. Yet it can be trained[citation needed], and achieved with various degrees of intensity or accuracy.

The human capacity to recognize the bodily feelings of another is related to one's imitative capacities, and seems to be grounded in the innate capacity to associate the bodily movements and facial expressions one sees in another with the proprioceptive feelings of producing those corresponding movements or expressions oneself. Humans also seem to make the same immediate connection between the tone of voice and other vocal expressions and inner feeling.

"A.W.E.S.O.M.E. Living…!"

~ a lesson from the "Get Out of Bed and Go to Work" Philosophy

<u>Your life can be AWESOME if you live in</u>:

Acceptance[2] (and Awareness of things as they truly Are)
Within (a qualifier that assumes genuine desire)
Expectation[1] (the one expectation is a desire to improve individually); of,
Self (and take the time to know yourself); and
Others (immerse yourself in loving relationships/organizations); with
Mutual (build a team by sharing openly and honestly)
Enthusiasm (Honor and be Inspired by your collective efforts)

Lon Kieffer, RN, BSN, MBA, NHA

Lon Kieffer, Author of "Get Out of Bed and Go to Work!", Speaker, Consultant and Expert on Workplace Culture Change and Generational Conflicts, gives seminars, keynote and plenary addresses, runs annual sales meetings, and provides Common Sense Consulting at:

Lon@LonKieffer.com

(302) 462-6748

www.LonKieffer.com

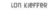

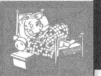

Join Lon in an amazing new and A.W.E.S.O.M.E. Adventure! There are 65.7 Million professional and non-professional Caregivers in the U.S. Today. Join the ONLY organization solely dedicated to understand and DEFEND Caregivers!

Go to www.defenderofcaregivers.com

A True Story... (an Excerpt from my book – "Get Out of Bed and Go to Work: Short Stories and Tall Tales of Awesome Living!")

I witnessed a miracle at WalMart. In line in front of me was a rough-looking kid wearing an over-sized leather jacket and baggy pants; he had a "doo-rag" on his head and iPod ear pieces in his ears-- you know the type. In front of him was a little old lady wearing a doo-rag of her own. A woman in her early 70's wearing a shower cap over some hair curlers-- you know the type...

I couldn't hear everything but gathered that the little-lady was late in preparing to have her family over for dinner; she would never be caught dead in public like this but needed some last minute things; on and on. The "thug" in front of me and directly behind her, heard none of this; but I could hear the thumping of his rap music leaking out and around his doo-rag.

This is when the problems started. Apparently the 70's-something lady in front didn't have cash with her-- only her checkbook; no wallet, no identification. The young pierced and tattooed, gum-chewing gal at the register (you know the type...) would not take her check without ID. I was late for an appointment and growing impatient (you know the type....) the "thug" was oblivious as he be-bopped along rhythmically slapping his thighs and "rubber-necking" his head and shoulders.

Before I could react it happened; there was nothing I could do!

The thug in front of me yanked the ear-plugs from under his doo-rag and in a loud abrupt voice said, "Lady!" (I braced myself, ready to pounce!) "You look honest; write the check out to me. I got this...." He then reached deep down into his baggy pants and pulled out his wallet from somewhere below his right knee and paid for that 70's-something lady's groceries with cash, and took her personal check.

It's A.W.E.S.O.M.E. to know that no matter how they may look; this next generation... THEY'VE GOT OUR BACK!

Made in the USA
Coppell, TX
15 May 2021

55751342R00075